REAL-WORLD NURSING SURVIVAL GUIDE:
IV THERAPY

REAL WORLD NURSING SURVIVAL GUIDE SERIES

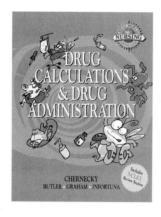

DRUG CALCULATIONS & DRUG ADMINISTRATION

CHERNECKY
BUTLER • GRAHAM • INFORTUNA

Includes NCLEX Review Section

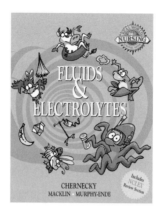

FLUIDS & ELECTROLYTES

CHERNECKY
MACKLIN • MURPHY-ENDE

Includes NCLEX Review Section

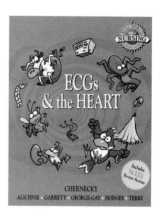

ECGs & the HEART

CHERNECKY
ALICHNIE • GARRETT • GEORGE-GAY • HODGES • TERRY

Includes NCLEX Review Section

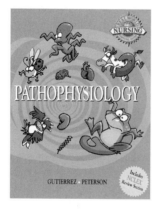

PATHOPHYSIOLOGY

GUTIERREZ • PETERSON

Includes NCLEX Review Section

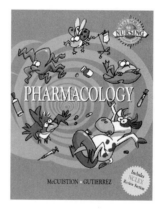

PHARMACOLOGY

McCUISTION • GUTIERREZ

Includes NCLEX Review Section

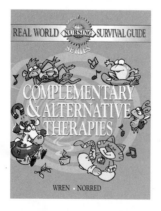

REAL WORLD NURSING SURVIVAL GUIDE SERIES

COMPLEMENTARY & ALTERNATIVE THERAPIES

WREN • NORRED

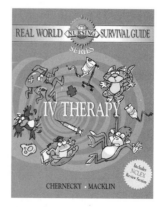

REAL WORLD NURSING SURVIVAL GUIDE SERIES

IV THERAPY

CHERNECKY • MACKLIN

Includes NCLEX Review Section

Real-World Nursing Survival Guide:
IV THERAPY

DENISE MACKLIN, BSN, RN, BC, CRNI
President, Professional Learning Systems, Inc.
Marietta, Georgia

CYNTHIA CHERNECKY, PhD, RN, CNS, AOCN
Professor, Department of Nursing Science
Medical College of Georgia, School of Nursing
Augusta, Georgia

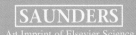

SAUNDERS
An Imprint of Elsevier Science

SAUNDERS

An Imprint of Elsevier Science

11830 Westline Industrial Drive
St. Louis, Missouri 63146

REAL-WORLD NURSING SURVIVAL GUIDE:
IV THERAPY

ISBN 0-7216-9778-X

NOTICE

Nursing is an ever-changing field. Standard safety precautions must be followed, but as new research and clinical experience broaden our knowledge, changes in treatment and drug therapy may become necessary or appropriate. Readers are advised to check the most current product information provided by the manufacturer of each drug to be administered to verify the recommended dose, the method and duration of administration, and contraindications. It is the responsibility of the licensed health care provider, relying on the experience and knowledge of the patient, to determine dosages and the best treatment for each individual patient. Neither the publisher nor the editor assumes any liability for any injury and/or damage to persons or property arising from this publication.

International Standard Book Number 0-7216-9778-X

Executive Vice President, Nursing and Health Professions: Sally Schrefer
Senior Acquisitions Editor: Robin Carter
Developmental Editor: Jamie Randall
Publishing Services Manager: Catherine Jackson
Design Manager: Amy Buxton
Cover Designer and Illustrators: Chris Sharp, Ted Bolte, GraphCom Corporation

Printed in the United States of America

Last digit is the print number: 9 8 7 6 5 4 3 2 1

About the Authors

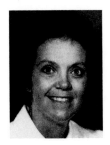 **Denise Macklin** is President and founder of Professional Learning Systems (PLS), Inc., and editor-in-chief of ceuzone.com, a continuing education Internet site. She is certified in IV therapy and adult/staff education. Denise has over 30 years of nursing experience with 17 years in the specialty of IV therapy. She was included in *Who's Who in Media and Communications 1998*. She is the recipient of the Suzanne Herbst award for vascular access and a research grant related to vascular access education from the National Institute for Nursing Research. Denise has lectured around the United States on a wide variety of IV therapy topics. She has published articles in various publications, including the *Journal of Intravenous Nursing, Journal of Vascular Access Devices, American Journal of Nursing,* and *Nursing Management and Dimensions of Critical Care*. She is a contributing author to *Saunders Manual of Medical-Surgical Nursing: A Guide to Clinical Decision Making* and co-author of the *Real World Nursing Survival Guide: Fluids & Electrolytes*. Denise's work includes extensive experience in the production of training videos for vascular access and interactive programs for medical manufacturers and the Centers for Disease Control and Prevention. PLS's videos, CD-i programs, and web CE offerings are being used to educate nurses worldwide.

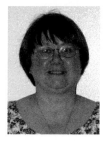

Dr. Cynthia Chernecky earned her degrees at the University of Connecticut (BSN), the University of Pittsburgh (MN), and Case Western Reserve University (PhD). She also earned an NCI fellowship at Yale University and a postdoctorate visiting scholarship at UCLA. Her clinical area of expertise is critical care oncology, with publications including *Laboratory Tests and Diagnostic Procedures* (fourth edition), *Advanced and Critical Care Oncology Nursing: Managing Primary Complications*, and several titles from the *Real-World Nursing Survival Guide Series*, including *ECGs & the Heart*, *Drug Calculations and Drug Administration*, and *Fluids & Electrolytes*. She is a national speaker, researcher, and published scholar in cancer nursing. She is also active in the Orthodox Church and enjoys life with family, friends, colleagues, and two West Highland white terriers.

Contributors

Troy E. Conner, BSN, CRNA
Tift Regional Medical Center
Tifton, Georgia

Kay Coulter, CRNI
Executive Director
Infusion Knowledge, Inc.
Clearwater, Florida

Corliss Derrick, MSN, RN
Instructor
Department of Adult Nursing
School of Nursing
Medical College of Georgia
Augusta, Georgia

Jim Leonard, CRNA, MN
DeKalb Anesthesia Associates, P.A.
Decatur, Georgia

Kathleen T. Mohn, MSEd, RN
Nurse Educator
Columbia Hospital Sunrise
Clinical Faculty Adjunct for Pediatrics & IV Therapy
Community College of Southern Nevada
Las Vegas, Nevada

Nancy Moureau
President
PICC Excellence
Orange Park, Florida

Faculty & Practitioner Reviewers

Jeanette Adams, PhD, CRNI, CS
Consultant
Coconut Grove, Florida

Patti Eisenberg, MN, CS
Medical-Surgical Clinical Nurse Specialist
Clinical Practice, Education and Research
Community Hospitals Indianapolis
Indianapolis, Indiana

Barbara Kiernan, PhD, APRN, BC
Assistant Professor
Medical College of Georgia
School of Nursing
Augusta, Georgia

Julie S. Snyder, MSN, RN, C
Adjunct Faculty
Christopher Newport University
Newport News, Virginia

Student Reviewers

FEATURED STUDENT REVIEWER

Jeffrey M. Waddell is a nontraditional student in the BSN program at Pittsburg State University in southeast Kansas. He graduated in May 2003 and plans to continue his education to earn his Master's degree and become a nurse practitioner with an emphasis in rheumatology while working either in a critical care setting or in an emergency department. He eventually plans to obtain a doctorate and teach in nursing. He started his professional years in 1995 as an EMT and eventually became a nationally registered and certified medical assistant, working for several years in the Kansas City area with a rheumatology practice. While in nursing school, he worked as a phlebotomist and an emergency room technician at Olathe Medical Center in Olathe, Kansas. In addition, he served as vice president of his nursing class and President of the Kansas Association of Nursing Students state executive board. In April 2002, he was elected to the National Student Nurses' Association (NSNA) Board of Directors and was appointed chair of the Membership Committee in addition to serving on the Breakthrough to Nursing committee and the Image of Nursing Committee. Jeff makes his home in Pleasanton, Kansas, with his wife Maggie and stepdaughter Kyla and looks forward to remaining active in nursing leadership and politics.

STUDENTS

Shelly Bryant
Valencia Community College
Orlando, Florida

Janice J. Carter, MLS
St. Louis University
School of Nursing
St. Louis, Missouri

Brandi E. Dingler
Medical College of Georgia
Athens, Georgia

Marni Dodd
Medical College of Georgia
Athens, Georgia

Debbie Eidam
Valencia Community College
Orlando, Florida

Jessica J. Fay
St. Louis University
School of Nursing
St. Louis, Missouri

Cindy Green, RN, CCE
Georgia League for Nursing
Columbus, Georgia

Lora L. Gregory
Valencia Community College
Orlando, Florida

Sarah Hackner
St. Louis University
School of Nursing
St. Louis, Missouri

Bridget Hamed, RN
Oakland Community College
Waterford, Michigan

Tricia B. Harrison
Beth-El College of Nursing and Health
    Sciences
University of Colorado at Colorado
    Springs
Colorado Springs, Colorado

Elizabeth Hunnicutt
Macon State College
Macon, Georgia

Amy M. Johnson
Beth-El College of Nursing and Health
    Sciences
University of Colorado
Colorado Springs, Colorado

Kelly Knox
Medical College of Georgia
Athens, Georgia

James C. Reedy, EMT
St. Louis University
School of Nursing
St. Louis, Missouri

Constance Riopelle
Oakland Community College
Waterford, Michigan

Raelynn Schafer, BS
Valencia Community College
Orlando, Florida

Kelly Swift
University of Iowa
Iowa City, Iowa

Sara Wyldwood
St. Louis University
School of Nursing
St. Louis, Missouri

Preface

Intravenous care is a major component of health care, and appropriate and research-based knowledge is essential to ensure positive patient outcomes. The area of intravenous nursing care is a specialty that includes both theoretical and clinical knowledge. Many changes in intravenous nursing care have occurred over the last decade; because of these changes, current nursing practice has been affected. We have written this book to meet the professional responsibility of educating nurses about the changes in intravenous nursing care. The primary purpose of *IV Therapy* is to offer an educational resource on the essentials of the principles of practice and nursing care associated with intravenous care. *IV Therapy* is written by nursing experts who have over 50 years of combined clinical experience in intravenous nursing care. Through our years in nursing practice, education, research, and as patients ourselves, we have become increasingly aware of many misconceptions and poor practice techniques associated with intravenous care, and we recognize that new practitioners need up-to-date information in the essentials of intravenous care. It is our hope that this book will enhance critical thinking, which is the hallmark of quality patient care.

IV Therapy begins by explaining the specifics of equipment and infusion regulation devices and is followed by principles of intravenous nursing care. We discuss the essentials of peripheral and central intravenous care to help decrease or avoid problems. The text includes specific chapters on different patient populations (pediatric, older adult) and areas of practice (community, home health care).

Once you understand the essentials of intravenous nursing care, you can more easily assimilate additional information regarding specialty care associated with intravenous therapy. Such special care areas include the emergency, critical care, and oncology departments. *IV Therapy* offers the essential foundations upon which you can build and thereby enhance intravenous nursing care to all of your patients. This text provides the foundational knowledge to go beyond the essentials into specialty care, if you desire.

IV Therapy includes many features in the margins to help you focus on the most important information needed to succeed in the classroom and in the clinical setting. **TAKE HOME POINTS** are composed of both study tips for classroom tests and "pearls of wisdom" designed to assist you in caring for patients. These points are drawn from our years of combined academic and clinical experience. Content marked with a **Caution** icon is vital and usually involves nursing actions that may have life-threatening consequences or those that may significantly affect patient outcomes. The **Lifespan** icon and the **Culture** icon highlight variations in treatment that may be necessary for specific age or ethnic groups. A **calculator** icon will draw your eye to important equations. A **Web Links** icon will direct you to sites on the Internet that will give more detailed information on a given topic. Each of these icons are designed to help you focus on real-world patient care, the nursing process, and positive patient outcomes.

We have also used consistent headings that emphasize specific nursing actions. **What It IS** provides a brief definition of the topic. **What You NEED TO KNOW** provides the explanation of the topic. **What You DO** explains what you do as a practicing nurse. Finally, **Do You UNDERSTAND?** provides questions and exercises that are both entertaining and useful to reinforce the topic's concepts. This four-step approach provides information and helps you learn how to apply this information to the clinical setting.

We hope this book will make a difficult topic easier and provide you with new insights and understanding of intravenous nursing care.

Denise Macklin, BSN, RN, BC, CRNI
Cynthia Chernecky, PhD, RN, CNS, AOCN

Acknowledgments

I would like to thank my colleague, mentor, and friend, Cynthia Chernecky, for her generosity of spirit and enthusiasm for life. Her support throughout the writing of this book, as well as during many other professional activities, have been invaluable to me. I would like to thank the contributing authors, especially Jeanette Adams, Nancy Moureau, and Kay Coulter, who have devoted their professional careers to the advancement of IV therapy education and for lending their special expertise to this book.

A special thanks for the never-ending encouragement, assistance, and friendship of my sister and partner Judith Carnahan. I would not have been able to complete this book or any of my many professional activities in research, authorship, and multimedia production without her.

I want to thank Robin Carter, Gina Hopf, Kristin Geen, Jamie Randall, and Dana Peick for all their patience, suggestions, and guidance. Their attention to detail has been invaluable to the development of this straightforward and easy-to-use book.

Finally, I would like to thank my husband, Dana, who has believed in me and understood the long hours, missed meals, and trips that were required to complete this book.

Denise Macklin

This book would not have been possible without personal dedication and a combination of professionalism and friendship. Such is the case with my co-author, Denise Macklin. We both have a passion for our profession, particularly the clinical and research sides, and know the glory of friendship. I also know that there is, through curriculum changes and threading of concepts in nursing curricula, the potential if not the actual loss of expertise in regards to intravenous nursing care. We have written this book to help students and practitioners take the information we have given and apply it to each individual patient. This book is also our way of hoping we do not lose the art and science of this aspect of nursing and can preserve the current knowledge for future nurses.

It is important that I truly recognize all the contributing authors who have given their time and expertise. I thank you from my heart for your dedication and caring. It is only a great work when everyone shares his or her expertise. We have done well!!!

This book is also the work of many who have supported me in my efforts as a nurse educator and researcher and, most importantly, as a daughter and friend. These beloved people are my mother Olga; Godmother Helen Prohorik; brother Richard; nieces Ellie and Annie; nephew Michael; cousins Paula Smart, Philip Prohorik, and Karyn Tarutis; Goddaughter Dawn Priscilla Payne; Godsons Jonathon Tarutis and Vincent Hunter; colleagues and friends Dr. Ann Marie Kolanowski, Dr. Joyceen Boyle, Dr. Katherine Maeve, Dr. Katherine Nugent, Dr. Linda Sarna, Dr. Jean Brown, Dr. Geraldine Padilla, Dr. Mary Cooley, Dr. Roma Williams, Dr. Leda Danao, Dr. Ruth McCorkle, Dr. Kathy Wren, Tim Wren, Pam Cushman, Kimberly Black, Tom Smart, Molly Loney, His Eminence Archbishop Dmitri of Dallas and the South in the Orthodox Church in America; Mother Thecla, the Abbess of Saints Mary and Martha Orthodox Monastery; Mother Helena; and Sister Seraphima.

I would also like to thank the publishing partners for their dedication to the profession of nursing and for blessing us with a wonderful group of colleagues, Robin Carter, Gina Hopf, Kristin Geen, Jamie Randall, and Dana Peick.

Dr. Cynthia (Cinda) Chernecky

Contents

1 Equipment and Infusion Regulation Devices

Top Bananas: Chapter 1 Overview

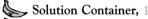

What IS a Solution Container?

Solution containers are materials that hold intravenous (IV) solutions and are categorized by their composition, either glass or plastic.

What You NEED TO KNOW

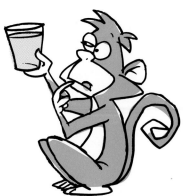

An understanding of how the fluid in different types of containers flows will help in selecting the appropriate administration sets to promote optimal function and minimize problems. The first system is "open"; it depends on air entering the container and pushing the fluid out. The second system is "closed," and it depends on atmospheric pressure.

1

Open
System
(Vented)

Closed
System
Soft Plastic
(Nonvented)

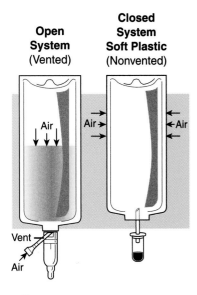

Vent

Air

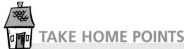

TAKE HOME POINTS

- Glass containers require a vented administration set.
- Glass containers are required for some fluids.

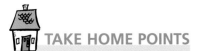

TAKE HOME POINTS

Soft, plastic containers use a non-vented administration set.

Open: Glass containers are rigid and vacuum sealed. Air must be allowed to enter the bottle to achieve a fluid flow. This feature means a vented administration, which allows air to enter through a filter into the solution, is required. Although glass containers are not commonly used today, they are used for infusates that cannot adapt to plastic bags because of incompatibilities with the chemicals or properties of plastic. Examples include lipids (when not in 3-in-1 total parenteral nutrition [TPN] solution) and nitroglycerin (glass required). There are several advantages to glass. Glass provides excellent visualization of the solution. It is easy to see particulate matter and the fluid level and to identify calibrations on the bottle accurately. Glass is inert so that it cannot react with the fluid contents. The disadvantages of a glass bottle are that it can break, it requires more space for storage and disposal compared with plastic, and its rubber septum is cored by the administration set spike during entry, which creates a potential for contamination.

Closed: The soft plastic bag uses atmospheric pressure pushing against the soft plastic to collapse the bag and force the fluid out. Because air entering the bag is not required, a nonvented administration set is used. This type of solution container is the most common type used today. The advantages of a plastic container are that it is lightweight, easy to store and dispose, does not break, is not sensitive to temperature fluctuation, and is not cored by the administration set spike during entry. The disadvantages are that plastic can be punctured, and some drugs can adhere to the plastic, thereby decreasing the amount of the drug received by the patient. Some plastic bags contain D_1 (2-elhylheryl) phthalate (DEHP) (a plasticizer that makes plastic soft and flexible), which can leach into or be degraded by the solution. The use of plastic bags is controversial with some medications (e.g., insulin, nitroglycerin, fat emulsions, lorazepam). The semirigid plastic containers contain no plasticizers, which eliminates compatibility problems, but they are bulky like glass containers. Semirigid plastic containers do not completely collapse as do plastic bags and leave about 50 ml of solution in the container when the infusion is complete. To eliminate this problem, use vented administration sets on semirigid plastic containers.

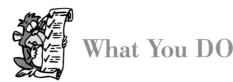

What You DO

Glass containers have an easily removable rubber disk that covers the rubber stopper. Once the disk is removed, the container must be used immediately. If the container has had an admixture added by the pharmacist, a new sterile cover will have been applied along with a label stating the additives. For stock solutions in plastic bags, the wrapper must be removed first. Pooling of fluid should not occur inside the wrapper. If pooling has occurred, do not use the solution.

Examine all containers for any defects. Examine the solution for clarity, precipitates, and discoloration. Check the expiration date on the label. If any problems are detected, label the container "contaminated" and return to central supply. Occasionally, small bubbles resembling champagne bubbles will be seen in a plastic bag that has been refrigerated. To eliminate these bubbles, shake the bag vigorously to move them toward the bottom of the bag. When spiking the bag, the bubbles will escape during the priming process. The time should be marked directly on a glass bottle. However, marking should be avoided with plastic containers because the ink from the marker can leach through the plastic into the solution. Tape the bag and then mark the tape. Some drugs are light-sensitive. These solution containers must be covered with a dark bag or aluminum foil during infusion. An example is nitroprusside sodium (Nipride).

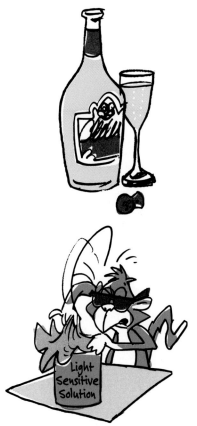

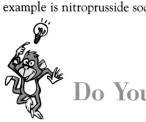

Do You UNDERSTAND?

DIRECTIONS: **Unscramble the words in parentheses to fill in the blanks.**

1. _____ containers are rigid and require vented administration sets. (*lsags*)

2. Glass enables the nurse to see through it clearly. The process of being able to see clearly through the glass is called _____. (*tailzunviosai*)

3. Soft _____ containers use a nonvented administration set. (*lstipac*)

Answers: 1. Glass; 2. visualization; 3. Plastic.

DIRECTIONS: **Place a "G" for glass container and a "P" for plastic container next to the type of drug to be administered in that container.**

4. _____ Single-dose lipids

5. _____ Normal saline

6. _____ Lorazepam

7. _____ Multivitamin

8. _____ 10 mg potassium chloride

9. _____ Morphine

10. _____ Nitroglycerine

DIRECTIONS: **Match Column A with Column B.**

Column A	Column B
11. _____ It uses a vented administration set.	a. Glass container
12. _____ It is used for nitroglycerin administration.	b. Plastic container
13. _____ It uses a nonvented administration set.	
14. _____ It is a lightweight container.	
15. _____ Accurate fluid levels are difficult to determine.	
16. _____ It is inert.	
17. _____ Rubber septum is cored by administration spike.	

DIRECTIONS: **Place a check mark next to the coverings that are typically used on light-sensitive medications.**

18. _____ a. Aluminum foil

_____ b. Alcohol-soaked gauze

_____ c. Toilet tissue

_____ d. Dark bag

_____ e. Clear plastic wrap

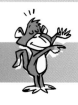

What IS an Administration Set?

Administration sets are kits that include IV tubing and associated parts. These sets are designed based on their usage. Administration sets vary in length and the size of the drip chambers. Some sets have two separate tubings. Each set is packaged individually and is labeled with the name, description, lot number, drops/ml, usage description, and the manufacturer's name. The types of administration sets are primary, secondary, metered-volume, and specialty.

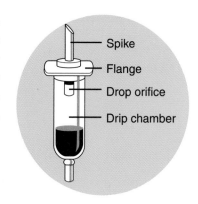

Spike
Flange
Drop orifice
Drip chamber

What You NEED TO KNOW

Administration sets include a spike, drop orifice, drip chamber, tubing, and clamp.

Spike: The spike pierces the solution reservoir. Spikes come with a vent (vented set), without a vent (nonvented set), or they are universal (can be both nonvented or vented). The sterile spike has a flange so that fingers do not touch the spike, thereby preventing contamination.

Drop orifice: The drop orifice is located at the top of the drip chamber. This orifice determines the size and shape of the drops. Calibrate these drops to calculate an infusion rate. There are two types of drop orifices: macrodrip (10 to 20 drops/ml) and microdrip (60 drops/ml).

Drip chamber: The drip chamber is the elongated, rigid section located just below the flange of the spike. The drip chamber has a hole at the top (drip orifice) and a hole at the bottom. The chamber is connected to the IV tubing.

Tubing: Tubing varies in flexibility, clarity, length, and internal diameter. Tubing is categorized by the internal lumen: standard, macro, or micro. Standard tubing is used for most infusions. Macro tubing has a larger channel and is usually stiffer compared with standard tubing. Macro tubing is used when high flow rates are required. A blood administration set is one example. Micro, or microbore tubing, has a smaller channel and thicker walls compared with standard tubing, which make it difficult to bend or stretch. Microbore tubing is commonly used for very low flow rates, such as continuous infusions of pain medications administered by an ambulatory pump.

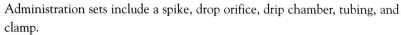

TAKE HOME POINTS

- With microdrip sets, the drops per minute are equal to the milliliters to be infused per hour. For example, a flow rate of 120 ml/hr equals 120 drops/min.
- Drop factors can be found printed on the boxes in which the administration sets are contained.
- The temperature and viscosity of the solution alters the size of the drop. Cold or thick solutions have larger drops than do warm or thin solutions.

 To calculate macrodrip sets, use the following equation:

Drops/ml is:

$$\frac{\text{Amount to be infused in 1 hour}}{60 \text{ minutes}} = \text{drops/min}$$

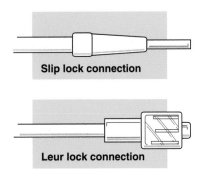

Slip lock connection

Leur lock connection

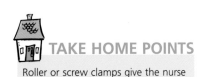
Tubing ends are configured with either a slip connection or a Leur connection. The slip connection slides onto the IV catheter and requires the use of some force. The Leur connection screws onto the catheter and requires no force. Nonpolyvinylchloride (non-PVC) tubing is available to be used with drugs that can interact with plasticizers. Paclitaxel (Taxol), an antineoplastic, is an example of a medication that requires non-PVC tubing.

Clamps: All clamps are categorized by design and consist of three types: slide, clip, screw, or roller (most common). Clamps alter the size of the internal channel of the tubing, enabling the nurse to regulate the fluid flow rate of the fluid. Slide or clip clamps are used for open or closed regulation and are found on secondary sets. Roller and screw clamps can be opened or closed in small increments to set a gravity flow rate.

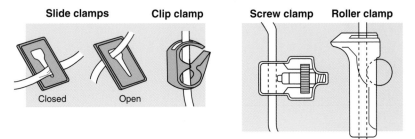

There are several different types of administration sets used to infuse medications and fluids: primary, secondary, metered-volume, and specialty.

Primary set: Primary sets are the main tubing attached to the primary solution (e.g., normal saline [NS], D₅NS, lactated Ringer's [LR] solution). The nonvented or universal design (using the nonvented option) is used with plastic bags. The vented configuration or the universal set (using the vented option) is used with glass bottles. Vented sets have an air filter that filters room air as it enters the fluid container. Primary sets have Leur connections, allowing them to be screwed onto a catheter securely. Primary sets also have **Y**-site connectors that are used to deliver different medications into the primary IV solution tubing. Typically, there are at least two **Y** connectors. One connector located on the top third of the tubing and one on the lower third. With primary tubing that is used with a secondary set, above the upper **Y** site, is a small disk called a back check valve. This valve allows fluid to flow from the primary container but prevents secondary medications from flowing back into the primary fluid container. The typical length of a primary set is 66 to 100 inches (165 to 250 cm). A back check valve may not be present on some pump tubing.

Secondary set: The secondary set is typically shorter than the primary tubing and is designed to attach to the primary set. To attach a secondary set to a primary set, some type of needleless system is needed. Secondary sets are used to deliver intermittent medications through the primary set. Secondary sets are commonly attached to the highest **Y** site on a primary set. However, some drugs will specify to be placed nearest the insertion site. Typical length of a secondary set is 32 to 42 inches (80 to 105 cm).

> ⚠️ **The secondary set must be attached to a primary set that has a back check valve. The valve prevents secondary solution from entering primary solution.**

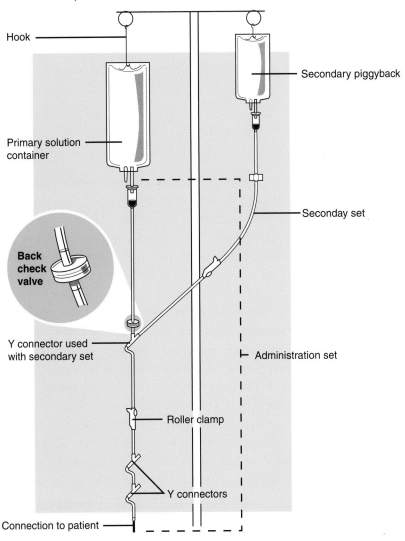

Hook

Secondary piggyback

Primary solution container

Seconday set

Back check valve

Y connector used with secondary set

Administration set

Roller clamp

Y connectors

Connection to patient

Metered-volume chamber set: These sets contain a flanged spike, then a roller clamp, followed by a large semirigid 10- to 50-ml chamber, then a filter, followed by a drip chamber, tubing, and a second roller clamp. These sets allow a specific, small amount of fluid to be filled in the chamber. The primary fluid roller clamp is then closed and the lower clamp is opened. These sets limit the total amount of fluid that can be administered.

Metered-volume chamber sets are typically used in infants, small children, and in critically ill adults (e.g., patients with heart failure or renal failure).

Tubing from one manufacturer's pump does not fit another manufacturer's pump.

• *Specialty sets:* Three examples of these sets are blood administration, non-PVC tubing, and pump-specific tubing.

  • *Blood administration sets:* These sets have two tubings each with a roller clamp located above the drip chamber. The first tubing will be attached to NS and the second tubing will be attached to the blood component.

  • *Non-PVC tubing and polyethylene-lined tubing:* The tubing may feel stiffer than does standard tubing and is used with paclitaxel, nitroglycerin, and lipids (when not in 3:1 TPN).

  • *Pump-specific tubing:* These sets are specific to a particular pump.

TAKE HOME POINTS

When spiking lipids in glass bottles, it is particularly important to place the glass bottle on the counter and spike downward while compressing the drip chamber. Once the bottle is spiked, raise the bottle and release the drip chamber. Lipids are extremely viscous and sticky. If lipids get into the air vent, the set is nonfunctioning, and a new set must be used.

⚠ **Do not use a needle inserted into the rubber stopper of a glass container to achieve a flow rate. The room air pulled into the bottle is not filtered and will contaminate the solution. Use a new administration set.**

What You DO

Choose the correct tubing for the specific needs of the prescribed infusion. Once the set is selected, open the set and slightly loosen the distal tubing end protector, but do not remove it. Some tubing has a vented cap and does not need to be loosened or removed during the priming procedure. Close all clamps on the tubing. Remove the spike protector. For glass bottles, it is easiest to stand the bottle on the counter. Squeeze the drip chamber (fingers behind the flange) and spike the bottle with a downward twisting motion. Once punctured, while maintaining the pressure on the drip chamber, the bottle is held upright and then the squeeze on the drip chamber is released. About one half of the drip chamber will fill with solution. This method prevents the air filter from getting wet and clogging. If the air filter gets clogged, a fluid flow will not occur. Hang the bottle on the pole and open the roller clamp **slowly** to begin the flow. This procedure minimizes the air being pulled into the tubing. As the descending fluid gets close to the distal end of the administration set, remove the protector cap and, with one hand on the roller clamp to regulate flow, carefully hold the tubing tip over a sink or garbage can to catch any escaping fluid. Close the roller clamp as fluid escapes through the tip and replace the protector cap. The tubing is now primed and ready to be connected to the patient.

With **plastic bags,** hold the IV spike flange (the bag will be lying flat on a surface), and remove the protective tab. Close all clamps on the tubing. Remove the spike protector, squeeze the drip chamber and spike using a twisting motion through the portal diaphragm. Be careful not to puncture the bag. Once the bag has been entered, raise the bag and then release the drip chamber. The drip chamber will fill half way. Hook the bag onto the IV pole, loosen the protector cap, and open the roller clamp **slowly** to prime the tubing. The primed tubing is now ready to be attached to the patient. The plastic bag can also hang on an IV pole, and the nurse can spike up into the bag. It is difficult to control the bag and the spiking procedure using this method. Lack of control means an increased potential exists for damaging the bag with the spike.

With **secondary tubing,** there are two methods for priming. The first method is similar to spiking either a glass bottle or plastic bag. The second method is called the "back fill" method. Spike the secondary container with the roller clamp closed, lower the secondary bag below the primary container, and open the clamp. The solution from the primary container will fill the secondary tubing first and then its drip chamber. Once the drip chamber is one-half full, the roller clamp should be closed and the secondary set should be hung onto the IV pole so that it is **higher** than the primary container. A hook is attached to the IV pole, and the primary solution is hung from the hook.

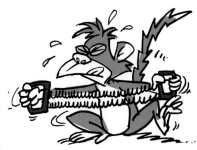

Open the secondary roller clamp completely and adjust the flow rate with the roller clamp located on the primary set. No drops will fall from the primary container's drip orifice. If the primary container continues to drip, lower the height of the primary container until the flow stops. Flow ceases from the primary container because of the pressure exerted by the secondary fluid on the back check valve. Once the secondary solution is administered, the secondary fluid pressure decreases, and the primary solution will again begin to flow.

With **metered-volume chamber sets,** close the roller clamp below the chamber. Spike the bag or bottle using the appropriate method and hang the bottle on the IV pole. Open the roller clamp above the chamber and squeeze the chamber. Fluid will fill the chamber. Additional squeezing motions may be needed to fill the chamber with the prescribed fluid completely. Open the roller clamp **below** the chamber and regulate the prescribed flow rate.

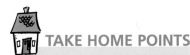

TAKE HOME POINTS

If the metered-volume chamber is allowed to empty completely, no fluid will be flowing, and the catheter can occlude. It is important to monitor metered-volume chamber sets closely.

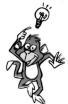

Do You UNDERSTAND?

DIRECTIONS: **Identify the following statements as** *true* **(T) or** *false* **(F).**

1. _____ The "spike" is the piece of the administration set that pierces the solution reservoir.
2. _____ The spike is not sterile.
3. _____ There are three types of drip orifices: macrodrip, minidrip, and milliondrip.

Answers: 1. T; 2. F; 3. F.

4. _____ In microdrip sets, the drops per minute are equal numerically to the milliliters to be infused per hour.

5._____ Cold solutions have larger drops than do hot solutions.

DIRECTIONS: **Answer the following questions.**

6. If a macrodrip (20 drops/ml) is prescribed at 100 ml/hr, then what are the drops per minute?

_____

7. If a macrodrip (10 drops/ml) is prescribed at 125 ml/hr, then what are the drops per minute?

_____

8. If the microdrip is prescribed for a flow rate of 50 ml/hr then what are the drops per minute?

_____

DIRECTIONS: **Label the following picture.**

9. _____

10. _____

11. _____

12. _____

DIRECTIONS: **Before each patient scenario, state if the patient needs a primary (P), secondary (S), or metered-volume chamber (M) set.**

13. _____ Mr. Goldberg is prescribed triple antibiotics IV piggyback (IVPB) after his tricuspid heart valve replacement.

14. _____ Miss Withington has chronic renal failure and has been prescribed the antibiotic gentamycin for a leg infection. The antibiotic is to be mixed in 40 ml of NS.

15. _____ Mrs. Zing is dehydrated and prescribed $D_5^{1}/_2NS$ at 200 ml/hr.

DIRECTIONS: **Fill in the blanks with the proper name of one of the six types of administration sets.**

16. I am the special type of administration set that has two tubings, one of which uses a bag of normal saline and a filter.

I am a _____ administration set.

17. I am a glass bottle of nitroglycerin that requires a

_____ or _____.

What IS an Add-On?

Add-ons are accessory equipment used with administration sets. Common examples include filters, extension tubing, connectors, stopcocks, and injection ports.

What You NEED TO KNOW

Filters remove both large (dust and rubber) and small particulates (bacteria and fungi) from the infusing solution. Filters are required with central venous, blood, intraspinal, and intraosseous fluid administrations. Selection is determined by pore size, pressure limitations, and solution. There are three types of filters: membrane, depth, and screen.

Membrane Filters

Another name for a membrane filter is end filter. This type of filter has a design similar to the grid on a piece of graph paper. The uniform squares are measured in microns and are either water loving or water hating (hydrophobic). The size of particulate that should be trapped determines the size of filter that is selected. All solutions can be filtered if the correct filter is selected. The common 0.22-micron filter cannot be used with some drugs because the drug is in suspension and the particles are too large to pass through. If a 0.22-micron filter is used, all of the medication will be filtered out. Lipids require a 1.2-micron filter; TPN 3:1 requires a 5-micron filter.

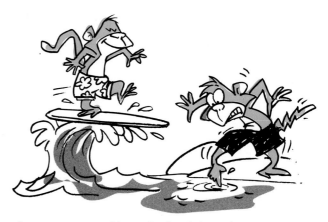

Drugs that can cause problems if infused through a 0.22-micron or smaller filter include the following:

- Penicillin G
- Potassium
- Cephalothin sodium
- Ampicillin sodium
- Mannitol
- Amphotericin B

The use of filters is required with TPN. Commonly, a 0.22-micron filter is used with TPN, and a 5-micron filter is used with 3:1 TPN. The use of filters on other solutions depends on institution policy. Filters are designed with air-eliminating vents that will allow air to escape. However, when a large air bolus enters a filter, this venting system is sometimes unable to clear the air. Because air is 5 microns in size, if the filter is filled with air, it will be blocked, and nothing will be able to flow through the filter.

Depth Filters

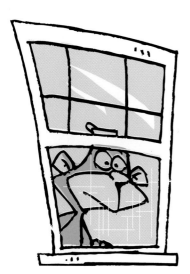

Depth filters absorb particles in several layers of randomly packed fibers comprising the filter media. The pore size is nonuniform and is rated according to the particulate size to be trapped. For example, leukocyte removal filters (LRFs) filter out any particles larger than 10 microns. Therefore this type of filter filters out the leukocytes but allows the smaller platelets to pass through.

Screen Filters

Screen filters look similar to window screens. The most common is seen in a blood administration set. The blood screen filter is 170 to 220 microns. This type of filter removes gross clots only. A microaggregate filter is also a screen filter, pore size 40 microns. This type of filter removes nonviable leukocytes, granulocytes, platelets, and fibrin strands. A micro-aggregate filter is used to prevent nonhemolytic febrile reactions and may decrease the sequelae known as adult respiratory distress syndrome (ARDS) .

Extension sets: Extension sets come in a variety of lengths and configurations based on the usage. These sets add length, clamping ability, or both and come in both macrobore and microbore configurations. The Centers for Disease Control and Prevention (CDC) does not recommend the routine use of extra tubing. Extensions should be used only for a specific purpose, such as the need for extra length when multiple IVs are required. Extensions should have a Leur connection.

Connectors: Connectors come in a variety of designs; some are added to the catheter to permit the infusion of 2 or 3 infusions (e.g., multiflow, Y). Some designs have Leur connections and may also include clip clamps. Some connectors are rigid (e.g., J-loop, U) and are added to form a rigid loop on peripheral catheters. Some connectors are soft, with slide or pinch clamps and possibly injection ports (e.g., T port).

Stopcocks: Stopcocks are special devices that determine the direction of solution flow; they come in three- or four-way configurations. A three-way stopcock allows two fluid paths to the patient, but only one can run at a time. A four-way stopcock allows two fluid paths to the patient either one at a time or both together, similar to a faucet that allows hot or cold or a combination of both to run through it at the same time.

Injection port systems: Injection ports are caps through which medications can be given quickly into the venous system. The capped catheter configuration permits IV access and intermittent use. In years past, the common cap was latex. However, today, needleless configurations are most prevalent. Be sure to identify an institution's needleless system. Needleless systems come in either positive pressure or nonpositive pressure configurations. Nursing interventions differ for each of the two systems. Nonpositive pressure systems require that the line be clamped before removing a syringe. Positive pressure systems require that the syringe first be removed and then the clamp be closed. If the wrong method is used, the cap can be damaged.

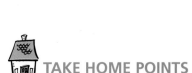

TAKE HOME POINTS
When using connectors, it is important to consider drug compatibilities.

TAKE HOME POINTS
Stopcocks are frequently used in intensive care settings.

What You DO

Determine the patient's current and near future IV needs before assembling the equipment to be used. All the equipment should come in sterile, intact packaging that is clearly labeled and includes an expiration date. Add

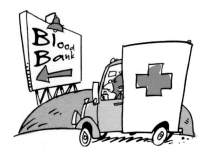

accessory equipment before priming the primary administration set. Common end filters have air vents that allow air in the tubing to escape during the priming procedure. If the filter becomes filled with air, gently tap the filter to force some air out of the vent. The motion will break the air lock and fluid will again flow. Make sure that all connections are tight. When administering blood through a Y-configured blood set, if the screen filter becomes clogged (flow will slow significantly or stop), close the blood clamp and open the saline clamp. Allow saline to flow into the chamber. This technique may open the system. If flow is achieved, close the saline, open the blood clamp, and attempt to resume infusion. If flow cannot be reestablished, the blood bag must be taken back to the blood bank. Do NOT spike the blood bag again with new tubing.

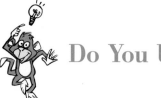

Do You UNDERSTAND?

DIRECTIONS: Complete the crossword puzzle on the following page.

Down

1. Common caps that use a needleless system are called injection

   _____.

2. Removes particles from infusion solutions.
6. These types include the multiflow, Y, J-loop, and U.

Across

3. These fats require at least a 1.2-μm filter.
4. This category of filter is common in blood administration sets.
5. Add-on that has three-way flow.
7. These sets add length or clamping ability.

DIRECTIONS: Identify the following statements as *true* (T) or *false* (F).

8. _____ Lipid infusions in glass bottles do not require air vents.
9. _____ A primary set is a type of add-on.
10. _____ Filters can remove dust, bacteria, fungi, and endotoxins.

DIRECTIONS: **Match the size of the filter required in Column A with the medications listed in Column B.**

Column A

11. _____ 1.2-μm filter
12. _____ 1.0-μm filter
13. _____ >0.22-μm filter
14. _____ 0.22-μm filter

Column B

a. mannitol
b. cephalothin sodium
c. cimetidine (Tagamet)
d. lipids

DIRECTIONS: **Unscramble the words in parentheses to fill in the blanks.**

15. A _____ comes in three-way and four-way types. *(ktocsocp)*

16. Accessory equipment used with administration sets includes _____. *(dasond)*

17. The three types of _____ are membrane, depth, and screen. *(selitfr)*

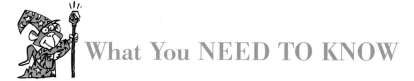

What IS an Infusion Regulation Device?

To deliver a prescribed infusion rate, the nurse must be able to regulate the flow. Several systems are available that enable regulation of fluid flow at various levels of accuracy.

What You NEED TO KNOW

Understanding the concept of pressure is important to understanding flow regulation. For fluid to flow, a pressure gradient must exist between the fluid container and the fluid destination (the patient). In the gravity infusion system, the pressure gradient is generated by the height of the bottle or bag. Rate is affected by the height of the solution container, patient activity, and the solution container's position relative to the patient's heart. This type of pressure does not vary as a result of the resistance that the system is generating by the contact of the fluid on the tubing and catheter as it flows. When an electronic pump is used, the force exerted by the pump generates the pressure gradient. The pressure exerted by the pump is related to the resistance the system is generating by the contact of the fluid on the tubing and catheter as it flows.

Three systems are used to regulate flow rate: gravitational, mechanical, and electronic.

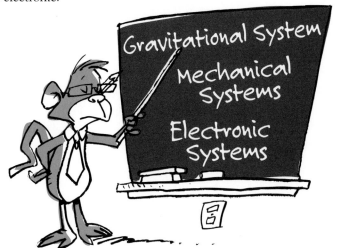

TAKE HOME POINTS

With an increase in central venous pressure (CVP) (> 6 mm Hg or 12 cm water) in conditions such as fluid overload, right-sided heart failure, and pulmonary hypertension, the use of gravity flow as a regulatory system is not recommended.

Gravitational System

The simplest method used to regulate flow is gravity. Placing the primary fluid 36 inches above the level of the patient's heart exerts about 1.3 pounds per square inch (psi). Because venous pressure ranges from 0.2 to 0.6 psi and central venous pressure ranges from 0.1 to 0.4 psi, gravity is sufficient to provide the necessary pressure gradient for fluid to flow into a person. Rate regulation is obtained by roller clamp manipulation. The advantage of gravity is low pressure exerted on the vein.

The disadvantages are lack of accuracy, free-flow prevention, and no rate change notification. Manual flow regulators are add-ons that are labeled with specific flow rates (e.g., Dial-A-Flow, Control-A-Flow). The flow rate is adjusted by turning the dial to the prescribed flow rate. However, the labeled rate may not be the true flow rate because of patient position, location of the catheter in the vein, and head height of the fluid container. Accuracy can vary from +/−10% to 25%.

TAKE HOME POINTS

Roller and screw clamps need to be repositioned on the IV tubing every 4 to 6 hours to enhance accuracy.

Mechanical Systems

Elastomeric pumps use a combination of atmospheric pressure and the addition of resistors added to the distal tip of the tubing to deliver a specific flow rate. A balloon inside a rigid container is filled with the solution (commonly antibiotics) to be infused. The balloon collapses over a specified period from 30 minutes to several days and is determined by the resistors located either on the distal end of the tubing or at the outlet of the container. These pumps are used in home care with the ambulatory patient. Rate accuracy can be altered when additional resistors are added to the system, such as infusing the solution cold instead of at room temperature.

- *Spring-loaded syringe pump:* With this device, a spring is stretched when the syringe is loaded. As the spring returns to its original nonstretched configuration, it applies pressure to the syringe plunger, causing fluid to flow.

- *Spring-coil container:* A stretched spring coil is surrounded by two disks. As the coil returns to a nonstretched configuration, it pulls the two disks together. These disks collapse the fluid container. The fluid is forced through device that produce resistance (restrictors).

Electronic Systems

Electronic devices were developed to improve accuracy, to prevent free flow, and to notify the caregiver of rate changes. Unlike gravity and mechanical systems, electronic systems require electricity, battery packs, or both. There are two types of systems: nonvolumetric and volumetric.

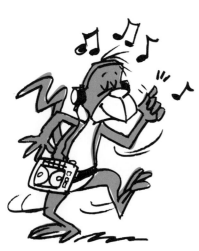

- *Nonvolumetric systems:* These devices, commonly called controllers, count drops using gravity as the pressure source. These devices are not pumps. Because gravity is the pressure source, resistors such as head height of the fluid container and the viscosity of the fluid can alter accuracy. Optimal head height for the fluid container is 36 inches above the patient's heart. These devices signal when the drop rate changes, altering the preset flow rate.

- *Volumetric pumps:* Volumetric pumps deliver a preset fluid rate over a specific period using constant force to overcome resistance in the IV line. These systems are highly accurate. Pumps require dedicated tubings or cassettes and are programmable, and many have additional program enhancements. Volumetric pumps come in ambulatory, patient-controlled analgesia (PCA), and single-dual-multichannel configurations. Pumps have preset psi limits (commonly 9 to 10 psi). When a pump is turned on, the pump takes an initial pressure reading; it then adjusts itself accordingly and sets the pressure limit slightly higher. This reading is the baseline pressure reading. When this baseline pressure limit is surpassed, the pump signals occlusion.

There are several different types of alarms: occlusion, air-in-line, and upstream alarms.

- **Occlusion alarm:** When a sensor identifies that the preset psi limit has been surpassed, an occlusion alarm will sound.
- **Air-in-line alarm:** When air bubbles pass through the pumping action, a sensor detects any air, and alarms will sound from the machine.
- **Upstream alarm:** This occurs when there is a problem between the solution container and the pump. The pump is unable to pull the required amount of fluid into the machine. The container may not be spiked correctly, the container may be empty, or a clamp above the machine has not been opened.
- **Other alarms:** Infusion complete, low battery or low power, not infusing, nonfunctional, and door open are other alarms that notify personnel that the pump is either not programmed correctly or that a system problem exists.

 ## What You DO

When hanging a primary solution, it should be elevated to 36 inches above the patient's heart. Remember, when the patient is sitting up or the bed has been elevated, assess the head height of the bottle and adjust if necessary. If the prescribed flow rate cannot be achieved, the resistance in the system may be high enough to prevent a sufficient pressure gradient to be achieved. Assess the system carefully. If no problems are identified, then elevate the height of the bottle slightly. The flow rate will increase when a required pressure gradient has been achieved. It is important to change the position of the roller clamp several times over an 8-hour period. The tubing under the roller clamp compresses and will alter the flow rate. Once the roller clamp is moved, squeeze the collapsed tubing; it will release and return to its original configuration. Not moving the roller clamp at least every 4 to 6 hours will result in gravity systems running slower than the prescribed flow rate.

It is important to understand how to use an electronic pump. Do not assume that all pumps are the same. Pumps are expensive, and assessing the patient's need for a pump is necessary. The following are some guidelines for pump use:

- All continuous fluids infusing through a central venous catheter or venous access device
- Pediatric and geriatric patients
- Fluid restricted patients (e.g., cardiac, renal)

 TAKE HOME POINTS

- Volumetric pumps are highly accurate in flow rates and very sensitive to flow problems in the patient or system.
- Each volumetric pump requires manufacturer-specific cassettes or tubing.

 On pumps that allow pressure limits to be set by the nurse, pressure limits should be maintained at a lower level in people with very friable veins, such as older adults.

TAKE HOME POINTS

Remember to open the clamp on the IV tubing before turning the electronic machine on, or it will signal an occlusion.

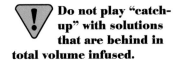 **Do not play "catch-up" with solutions that are behind in total volume infused.**

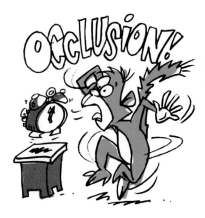

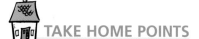

- TPN/HPA (total parenteral nutrition/hyperalimentation)
- Fluids requiring accuracy (e.g., heparin, aminophylline, insulin, pitocin, magnesium sulfate, chemotherapy, narcotics, sedatives, tissue plasminogen activator [tPA], vasoconstrictors, antiarrhythmic, antihypertensive, potassium bolus, solutions with more than 40 mEq/L potassium)

When pumps signal an "occlusion," this does not necessarily mean the catheter is occluded; it means that the maximum pump pressure limit has been met. The entire system should be investigated using the following checklist:

1. Is the IV catheter patent? Does it seem to be clotted off?
2. Is the IV site dressing too tight?
3. Are there signs of infiltration? Is the skin around the site puffy or red? Does the patient complain of site pain or discomfort?
4. Is the IV catheter kinked off? Recheck site placement.
5. Was a filter added to the line setup? Is it patent?
6. Has the rate been dramatically increased?
7. Has extension tubing been added?
8. Has the viscosity of the IV fluid changed?
9. Were additional infusion devices or syringe pumps added down line that might affect downstream baseline resistance?
10. What size IV catheter is being used?

When resetting pumps after an occlusion alarm, wait about 1 minute. This length of time will allow the pump to recalibrate at the new level. Make sure the IV catheter is immobilized, the dressing is secured, and there is a stress-prevention loop on the tubing. With planning and proper care, it is less likely that the patient will experience problems with IV infusions.

TAKE HOME POINTS

IV pumps do not cause infiltrations, nor can they detect them. Nursing care requires frequent visual inspection of an IV administration site.

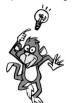

Do You UNDERSTAND?

DIRECTIONS: **Fill in the blanks to complete the statement.**

1. The three systems used to generate flow rates in an IV solution are

   _____, _____,

   and _____.

2. Gravity systems can change flow rates caused by three changes. These are changes in patient _____, location of

   _____, and _____

   of container.

DIRECTIONS: **Match the infusion system in Column A with the aspects of the system in Column B. Consider more than one aspect from Column B for each system.**

Column A

3. _____ Gravity system

4. _____ Mechanical system

5. _____ Electronic system

Column B

a. Disadvantage of free flow prevention

b. Uses atmospheric pressure and resistors

c. Requires electricity or battery

d. Simplest method to regulate flow

e. Type is a spring loaded syringe pump

f. Has a balloon inside a rigid container

g. Programmable pump that is highly accurate

DIRECTIONS: **Before each of the following conditions, place either an "O" for occlusion, an "A" for air-in-line, a "U" for upstream alarm, or an "OA" for other alarms to identify the type of alarm that will sound under the following conditions.**

6. _____ Stroke volume cannot be met because the container is not spiked correctly.

7. _____ Large champagne-type bubbles pass through the sensor.

8. _____ psi limit is surpassed because of a kink in the IV tubing.

9. _____ Low battery light is flashing on the IV machine.

DIRECTIONS: **Place a check mark next to the circumstances when an occlusion alarm would sound on an electronic IV pump.**

10. _____ a. IV dressing is too tight.

_____ b. IV is clotted.

_____ c. Air is in the IV line.

_____ d. Extension set is kinked.

_____ e. A medication given through a secondary set has finished infusion.

_____ f. The IV site is infiltrated.

Answers: 3, a, d; 4, b, e, f; 5, c, g; 6, U; 7, A; 8, O; 9, OA; 10, a, b, c, f.

CHAPTER

2 Principles of Peripheral Venous Therapy

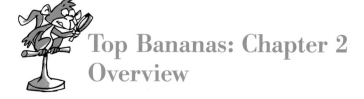

Top Bananas: Chapter 2 Overview

Selection Process, 30
Local Anesthesia, 41
Insertion Procedure, 45
Applying the Dressing, 52
Flushing Procedure, 55
Removal Procedure, 57
Documentation, 59
Patient Education, 61

Peripheral venous therapy is the infusion of intravenous (IV) solutions into a peripheral vein by means of a catheter. To place a catheter in a peripheral vein successfully, the nurse must understand how to do a venous assessment, how to select the appropriate vein and a suitable catheter, and the steps of the insertion process. Once venous access is obtained, successful stabilization and maintenance are important if the catheter is going to remain in place and free of complications until the end of therapy or routine rotation to a new site is required.

What IS IV Assessment?

Patient assessment associated with IV therapy is a complex process that includes collecting data from the patient's chart and the patient and then synthesizing this information with knowledge of pharmacology, fluid and electrolytes, anatomy, and physiology. Patient assessment is central to successful venipuncture. A thorough assessment enables the nurse to develop a plan of care that will facilitate positive patient outcomes and minimize complications.

What You NEED TO KNOW

It is important to know that there are several factors that affect successful peripheral IV therapy, including length of therapy, patient age, patient diagnoses, allergies, and type of therapy.

Length of therapy: Central to successful catheter selection is identifying the length of time the patient will require IV therapy. This period includes how long the current therapy will be, such as antibiotics for 3 days, and what the projected IV needs are, such as monthly chemotherapy infusions for 6 months. Duration is divided into three types:

- *Short term:* Less than 2 weeks
- *Intermediate:* 2- to 4-week course of therapy
- *Long term:* Greater than 4 weeks (either continuous or intermittent)

If the one-time needs of the patient are going to extend greater than 1 week, or if there are many anticipated treatments expected in the future, then an intermediate vascular-access device or a long-term vascular-access device may be considered.

Patient age: Skin consistency, vessel elasticity, fluid balance, and muscle mass differ with age, especially with the pediatric or geriatric patient. These differences affect site preparation, catheter selection, vein visualization and stabilization, catheter stabilization, dressing management, and fluid administration.

Patient diagnoses: Patients with chronic diseases and certain surgical procedures have altered venous access.

- *Heart disease:* Increased potential for venous spasm may occur that results in veins collapsing during venipuncture. The presence of edema can make locating a vein difficult.

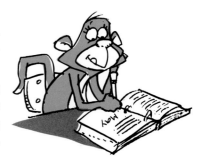

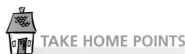
TAKE HOME POINTS

The average chemotherapy patient has a venous-access device for about 2 years.

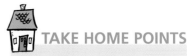
TAKE HOME POINTS

It is important to identify not only the current needs of the patient but also the long-term requirements.

Older adults have decreased vessel elasticity, and pediatric persons have decreased developed muscle mass.

- *Diabetes:* The walls of the veins may be thicker. Hyperglycemia activates plasma proteins that increase vasoconstriction. Because of increased platelet aggregation, the potential for catheter occlusion is increased. The presence of peripheral neuropathy in the hands limits the patient's ability to feel tenderness at the insertion site or the skin over the catheter track. This lack of feeling limits the patient's ability to acknowledge early symptoms of phlebitis or infiltration to the nurse.
- *Renal disorders:* Patients may have shunts or may need shunts in the future, placing limitations on which arm can be used for venipuncture.
- *Diseases requiring chronic steroid use:* Examples include chronic obstructive pulmonary disease (COPD), lupus, arthritis, sarcoidosis, and connective tissue diagnoses. With long-term steroid use, skin and veins become fragile, which increases the potential for skin tears, bruising, and infiltration. Additionally, the use of steroids delays the symptoms of phlebitis.
- *Immunodeficiency diseases:* Examples include cancer, human immunodeficiency virus (HIV), and Crohn's disease. Signs of phlebitis may not be seen because of delayed onset, and the response to infection is also slowed. An elevated temperature of 101° F (38.2° C) may be the only sign of severe infection. The usual practice of not rotating a catheter because a sign of phlebitis is not present should be avoided in this population.
- *Surgical procedures:* Major upper extremity vascular surgery, mastectomy, arteriovenous graft may also produce altered venous access.

Allergies: Allergic reactions may be caused by skin preparations, catheter material, and latex.

Latex allergy risk factors are related to increased exposure:
- Multiple abdominal or genitourinary tract surgery (e.g., for spina bifida)
- Frequent urinary catheterizations
- Nursing, medical, and dental professional's extensive use of latex gloves
- Food allergies to bananas, avocados, tropical fruit, kiwi, or chestnuts
- History of allergies or asthma
- Female

Type of therapy: The type of therapy that is prescribed for the patient influences the size of the catheter and the vein selection. Drugs and solutions can be highly caustic to the vein. Proper hemodilution is important to prevent the drugs from burning the vein wall (chemical phlebitis). To maintain potency, reconstituted drugs require a certain pH range. For example, the greater the solution pH and/or osmolarity (number of solutes in a solution) or the greater the difference between normal blood pH (7.4) and osmolarity (290 mOsm/L) is, the greater the potential for phlebitis will be.

TAKE HOME POINTS

Assess platelet count and the use of anticoagulants before IV insertion to determine potential for bleeding and hematoma formation.

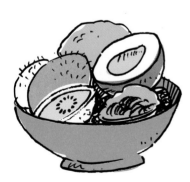

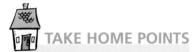

TAKE HOME POINTS

Risk for phlebitis increases as the solution deviates from a pH of 7.4 and an osmolarity of 290 mOsm/L.

What You DO

Laboratory values: Implement culture and sensitivity (C & S) laboratory tests before starting any IV antibiotics. If antibiotic therapy is begun before the C & S, the culture may not grow the culprit organism, and the C & S laboratory tests will be misleading. Have laboratory tests completed for electrolytes (sodium [Na^+], potassium [K^+], chlorine [Cl^-]) before beginning IV solutions containing electrolytes to have a baseline electrolyte level. This level is important in determining how much and which electrolytes to replace. Review serum blood urea nitrogen (BUN) and creatinine values to assess the patient's renal function. Renal function is associated with fluid homeostasis. Poor renal function can result in fluid overload. Review platelet count, International Normalized Ratio (INR), prothrombin time (PT), and partial thromboplastin time (PTT) laboratory results to assess the patient's bleeding potential. Bleeding potential will affect potential hematoma formation during venipuncture.

IV therapy history: Ask the patient about his or her experience with IV therapy. Prior IV procedures can limit the number and quality of accessible veins. Some questions to ask include the following:

- What IV drugs have you had in the past?
- How long ago did you have IVs?
- Did you have IV therapy in the hospital or at home?
- How often was the medication given?

Ask about oral (PO) medications, including both prescription and over-the-counter medications because these drugs may affect the venipuncture procedure. For example, if the patient is taking Coumadin or aspirin, care must be taken to prevent hematoma formation during insertion (tourniquet application should be loose to prevent the vein from bursting with catheter penetration) or bruising from occurring with catheter insertion or removal (direct pressure should be used over the IV site for 3 to 5 minutes after catheter removal).

Absorption of prescribed IV medications may be altered or incompatible with other medications the patient is taking. Before using an iodine-based skin preparation, ask if the patient is allergic to iodine or shellfish, and, if so, use a noniodine-based skin preparation. It is important to review all of the

TAKE HOME POINTS

Patients receiving Plavix, aspirin, NSAIDs,Coumadin, or heparin have an increased potential for hematoma formation during venipuncture.

patient's allergies, including food allergies, for hints that may predispose latex allergy. Latex is present in a variety of equipment related to IV therapy, including the following:

- Tourniquets
- Adhesive tape, Band Aids
- Blood pressure cuffs
- Disposable syringes
- Diaphragm on vials
- Gloves
- Injection caps
- Injection ports

Alternative latex-free products will have to be used with latex-allergic patients.

Physical assessment: Once the chart review is completed and all necessary laboratory tests have been drawn, and after an IV history has been determined, the nurse needs to complete a physical assessment of the patient.

Skin: The presence of adipose tissue or edema (or both) can make venous assessment difficult and alter the angle necessary for penetration during insertion. The color of the skin helps determine perfusion. Pale, gray, or cyanotic skin tone is reflective of poor perfusion. Good peripheral circulation is necessary to achieve adequate hemodilution, drug circulation, and absorption. Assess hydration status. If the patient's hand is elevated for 3 to 5 seconds, the veins should empty. In circulatory overload, hand veins will continue to be clearly visible. Dehydration can make venous distention difficult to achieve. Gently pinch the skin and then release it, noting the ability of the skin to return to its original shape. Older, dehydrated, and cachectic patients have loss of tissue elasticity. Loss of tissue elasticity can make vein stabilization difficult. Assess for areas of bruising, rashes, or breaks in the skin. These areas should be avoided when choosing a site for venipuncture.

Identify any conditions involving limb restrictions, such as:

- Motor or sensory function (patient might be unable to feel pain or discomfort of the IV)
- Cerebrovascular accident (CVA, stroke) (patient might be unable to feel pain or discomfort of IV)
- Mastectomy (possible compromised venous or lymph system functioning)
- Arteriovenous (AV) shunt and graft (venous system already in use)

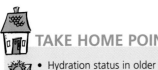

TAKE HOME POINTS

- Hydration status in older adults can be assessed by pinching the skin of the forehead or sternum, not the arm or hand. However, this indicator of hydration status may be unreliable.
- With thin skin, care must be taken with tourniquet application, as well as vein stabilization, dressing selection, and dressing removal, to avoid tearing the skin.

IV catheters should not be placed in arms with these limitations. Identify mobility requirements, such as hand dominance, the use of walkers, over-the-bed trapeze, and crutches. If the patient is restricted to bed, determine how the patient is moved to a chair or transported for tests. Extremity restrictions affect all aspects of the venipuncture. Placing catheters in areas of flexion, pressure, or locations that can be easily snagged increases the potential for catheter occlusion, dislodgment, or damage.

Mental status: Confused or combative patients present special problems with site selection, vein stabilization, insertion, and dressing maintenance. Restraints should not be placed over a venipuncture site, but rather, distal to the site. The anxious patient is at high risk for venous spasm. Venous spasm can cause a large visible vein to disappear when accessed or make catheter advancement into the vein impossible. Venous spasms can be so severe that the catheter can be pushed back out of the vein.

Transcultural barriers: It is important to have patient cooperation during the venipuncture procedure. Transcultural barriers can affect the level of cooperation. Language is the biggest barrier. Identify a bilingual person to assist in all phases of the venipuncture procedure. Other transcultural barriers include:

- Communication style (nonverbal, touch)
- Beliefs about illness
- Beliefs about why one is ill
- Beliefs about prevention of illness
- Religion
- Space (social distance)
- Gender issues

Identify the patient's support group that will be helping with care and providing emotional support. The caregiver's assistance may make the difference between success and failure.

With the alert, cooperative patient, it is important to seek patient preferences and incorporate these preferences into the plan of care. Patients can be highly needle-phobic or sensitive to pain. Response to fear and pain can cause venous spasm.

Hand dominance is important. Placing an IV in the nondominant extremity is preferable. However, if the patient is having surgery, it is preferable to place the IV in the dominant side first (if IV location is not specified in the physician prescription) so that when the patient is alert, the IV rotation (to a smaller gauge size) will be moved to the nondominant hand.

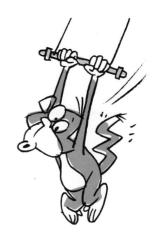

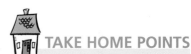

TAKE HOME POINTS

Any limb with restrictions should not be used for routine venipuncture.

Assessment of potential transcultural barriers will aid in obtaining positive outcomes related to IV insertion.

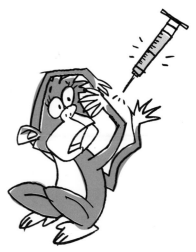

TAKE HOME POINTS

Large gauge catheters used for surgery should be rotated to smaller gauge catheters when therapy permits to minimize the potential for phlebitis (see Chapter 3).

At the completion of the assessment process, the overall location for IV placement, the gauge size of the catheter required for the prescribed therapy, the need for assistance with the venipuncture procedure, and the factors that can increase the potential for complication occurrence should have been identified. Then a plan of care that will minimize the impact of these factors and result in high patient satisfaction should be developed.

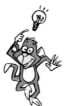

Do You UNDERSTAND?

DIRECTIONS: Provide the answer(s) to the following question.

1. Which of the following areas are needed to best help the nurse perform a thorough assessment of a person who is about to obtain an IV? (*Circle correct responses.*)

Anatomy   Physiology

Fluids and electrolytes   Pharmacology

Electrocardiogram (ECG) interpretation   Botany

DIRECTIONS: Match the term associated with the length of IV therapy in Column A to its definition in Column B.

Column A   Column B

2. _____ Short-term   a. 2 to 4 weeks

3. _____ Intermediate   b. Greater than 4 weeks

4. _____ Long-term   c. Less than 2 weeks

DIRECTIONS: Write the name of the chronic disease that alters venous access under the physiologic statement associated with the disease.

5. This disease increases venous spasm, and the presence of edema makes locating a vein difficult.

_____

6. This disease activates plasma proteins that increase vasoconstriction in response to hyperglycemia.

_____

7. With this group of chronic diseases, the skin and veins become fragile, resulting from long-term steroid use that is necessary to decrease pulmonary symptoms.

    _____

8. In this category of diseases, the response to signs of infection and phlebitis is usually slow.

    _____

DIRECTIONS: **Provide the correct answer(s) to the following question.**

9. People who are allergic to latex should avoid which of the following foods? (*Circle the correct answers.*)

bananas	beans	broccoli
kiwi	avocados	beef
chestnuts	bacon	potato chips

DIRECTIONS: **Match the laboratory test that should have been performed before the treatment listed.**

Laboratory Test   Treatment

10. _____ C & S   a. Begin normal saline IV

11. _____ Serum creatinine   b. Begin antibiotic therapy

12. _____ Platelet count   c. Renal disease treatment

13. _____ Serum Na$^+$ d. Treatment for bleeding

DIRECTIONS: **Provide answers to the following instruction and question.**

14. Name five medications that should be assessed if the nurse wants to know if the patient is likely to develop a hematoma after venipuncture.

    _____   _____

    _____   _____

    _____

15. Which of the following equipment that is related to IV therapy may contain latex and should therefore be avoided in individuals with latex allergies? (*Circle all answers that apply.*)

Blood pressure cuff	Stethoscope
Tourniquet	Disposable syringe
Hypoallergenic tape	Injection port

16. Which hydration status (overhydration or dehydration) makes venous distention difficult to achieve?

_____

17. Limb mobility restriction can be caused by a number of factors and can affect IV therapy. Which factors can cause restriction of limb mobility?

_____
_____
_____
_____
_____

What IS the Selection Process?

Before performing a venipuncture, the nurse must select not only a vein, but also the appropriate catheter for insertion. In addition to selecting a vein for the immediate infusion, an inventory of potential sites should be made to determine (in the best- and worst-case scenarios) if the end of therapy can be achieved using the short-term peripheral route. The nurse integrates information about anatomy, physiology, and the principles of physics to complete all aspects of the selection process successfully. This knowledge will help in the development of an IV plan of care that will minimize complication occurrence, develop appropriate interventions to treat complications when they occur, and alter the plan of care to prevent further problems.

What You NEED TO KNOW

Understanding the anatomy of peripheral vasculature helps in choosing an insertion site that will minimize IV complications. (See Chapter 3.) The vein wall is composed of three layers: tunica intima, tunica media, and tunica adventitia.

• _Tunica intima_ is the innermost layer of the vein and is divided into three layers. The innermost layer is composed of a single layer of flat epithelial cells.

These tightly packed cells provide a smooth surface, which reduces resistance to flowing blood. Endothelial cells produce prostacyclin, which inhibits platelet aggregation. Behind this layer is the subendothelium where substances are released that enhance clot formation. Damage to the single layer of endothelial cells of the intima initiates an inflammatory response.

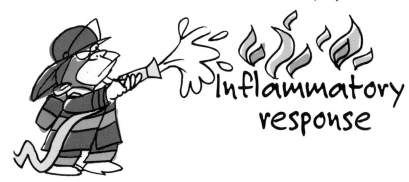

Platelets adhere to the damaged areas. The clotting cascade and the fibrinolytic system are initiated. The opposing systems of the endothelial cells that line the vein and the subbasement endothelial cells allow thrombus formation to aid vein wall healing and thrombus dissolution as healing occurs. The outer layer of the tunica intima is an elastic membrane that separates the intima from the middle vein layer.

- *Tunica media* contains smooth muscle and elastic tissue and is sensitive to pressure changes, temperature, and trauma. The smooth muscle can contract and can also shorten, causing the vein to become progressively stiffer and less compliant. This state is experienced with second venipuncture attempts. The vein feels tougher and is more difficult to penetrate. This layer causes venous distention. With prolonged distention, the smooth muscle causes the vein to flatten (stress-relaxation phenomenon).

- *Tunica adventitia* is the outer layer and is made up of connective tissue that supports the vessel, sympathetic nerves that maintain vasomotor tone (venous pressure), and blood vessels (vasa vasorum) that nourish the vein.

- *Valves* are semilunar folds that assist with blood return to the heart; they occur throughout the venous tree, most notably at a bifurcation, and are visible as bulges when a tourniquet is applied.

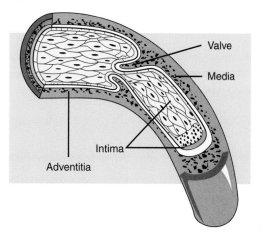

Common veins used for peripheral venipuncture are found in the hands and forearms. Veins increase in size with increasing proximity to the heart. Peripheral veins of the hand and lower forearm are small, major upper arm veins double in size, and the superior vena cava is twice as large as are the major vessels of the upper arm.

- *Metacarpal:* Dorsal aspect of hand

  Advantage: Easy visualization, easy to palpate, lowest site available, has +35 mm Hg hydrostatic pressure

  Disadvantage: May be difficult to stabilize, limits mobility, smaller than veins higher on the forearm

- *Basilic:* Inner aspect of forearm (little finger side) from wrist to shoulder (the largest vein)

  Advantage: Easy to palpate and visualize

  Disadvantage: Location makes venipuncture more difficult (difficult for the patient to see)

- *Cephalic:* Radial side of arm (thumb side) wrist to shoulder

  Advantage: Easy to see, palpate, and stabilize

  Disadvantage: Joint movement may increase potential for vein wall trauma

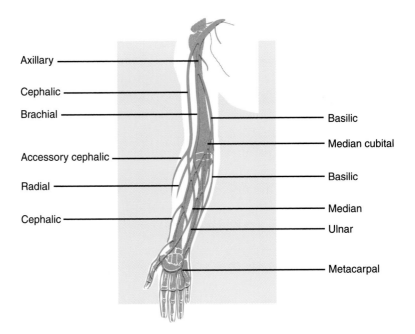

- **Accessory cephalic:** Branches of cephalic vein along radial bone
  Advantage: Easy to visualize and palpate
  Disadvantage: Valve present at junction of cephalic vein
- **Median:** Ventral forearm above palm, joins basilic vein slightly below the antecubital fossa on the medial aspect of the forearm
  Advantage: Easy to visualize and palpate
  Disadvantage: Increased pain sensation with venipuncture
- **External jugular:** Used in emergency situations by specially trained personnel because it is easy to access (catheter placed in this site is usually removed when the patient is stabilized and an alternative site is found)
  Advantage: Because of its large size and close proximity to the heart, it can be palpated and accessed during periods of stress when the peripheral veins are constricted
  Disadvantage: Dressings are difficult to maintain with this site; neck movement can affect flow rate

Veins of the feet can also be used for venous access. The use of feet veins in adults is limited because of potential for decreased circulation and loss of mobility. Feet veins in adults are usually used for venograms of the legs with a physician's prescription.

Physical Principles of Flow

To select the appropriate catheter for insertion and successfully troubleshoot problems when they arise, it is necessary to understand some basic physical principles of flow or how fluids get from one place to another. The IV solution is able to flow through the tubing, the IV cannula, and into the vein as a result of the relationship between resistance and pressure. Resistance is anything that impedes flow. As resistance increases, flow rate decreases. Fluid viscosity, catheter length, and internal diameter are the major resistors to flow.

- **Viscosity:** Viscosity is defined as the thickness or gumminess of a fluid. Principle: double the viscosity, and the flow rate will be halved. Temperature directly affects fluid viscosity. The colder the fluid is, the thicker it is. This characteristic is seen with blood infusions. When the infusion rate for blood is initially calculated and then not recalibrated over time, the infusion rate increases, and the blood will infuse faster than is anticipated, largely because the blood warms and thins. As blood thins, the infusion rate increases.

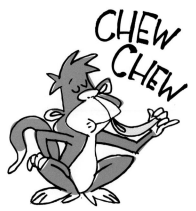

Same-Gauge Catheter

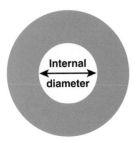

Nonthin wall

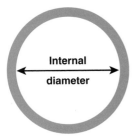

Thin wall

- **Length:** Principle: double the length, and the flow rate will be halved. Long catheters have slower infusion rates than do short catheters. Adding long lengths of tubing decreases the flow rate.
- **Internal diameter:** Diameter is the distance from one inside edge of the catheter lumen to the opposite side. Principle: double the diameter of the internal diameter, and the flow rate will be increased to the mathematical power of four.

Catheter wall thickness determines the internal diameter of the catheter. Peripheral catheters can be either thin wall or nonthin wall. This feature can be accomplished by design or by material. Peripheral catheters are made of either Teflon or polyurethane. Polyurethane catheters are always thin wall. Teflon catheters are commonly nonthin wall catheters. Therefore, catheters with the same gauge can have different flow rates, depending on catheter design and material.

The 24-gauge thin wall catheter has approximately the same flow rate as does the 22-gauge nonthin wall design. The 18-gauge thin wall has the same flow rate as does the 16-gauge 5-inch catheter.

Comparison of Thin Wall versus Nonthin Wall Catheters

GAUGE	THIN WALL (INSTYE POLYURETHANE)		NONTHIN WALL (ANGIOCATH) TEFLON	
	Length	Flow (ml/min)	Length	Flow (ml/min)
24	1/2"	24.4	3/4"	16.4
22	1"	36.4	1"	27.6
18	1 1/4"	107.9	1 1/4"	85.2
16	2"	204.7	5"	108.0

TAKE HOME POINTS

- The higher the numeral, the smaller the gauge size (e.g., a 16-gauge catheter is larger than a 20-gauge catheter).
- Gauge size denotes the circumference of the catheter and is standardized.
- Viscosity, length, and internal diameter influence flow rate and are known as resistors.

Peripheral catheters reside in veins and depend on the flow of blood around them to dilute the solution or medication (infusates) and provide a buffer between the catheter and the vein wall.

Fluid follows the path of least resistance. When the catheter/vein ratio is poor, or when a small tributary vein is accessed, the flowing blood will bypass the vein for another vein with an unrestricted lumen. The accessed vein has a much lower blood flow, preventing hemodilution and catheter buffer.

Catheter Configuration

To select the appropriate catheter, it is important to be able to identify the different configurations that are available.

- **Winged:** Commonly known as a "butterfly" catheter, this peripheral catheter consists of a stainless steel needle with soft pliable wings and an attached short-type of extension tubing. A butterfly is commonly used for blood draws and single dose, IV push medication. Dwell time is recommended for 1 to 2 hours. Although easy to insert, the biggest disadvantage with butterflies is that they require an arm board if used for short infusions; their stiffness increases the potential for infiltration. For this reason, butterflies should not be used with uncooperative patients or continuous infusions.

Winged Catheter

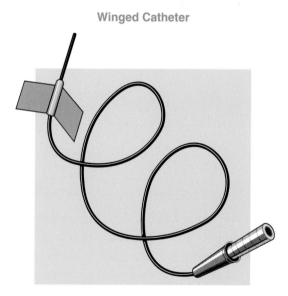

Over-the-Needle Catheter

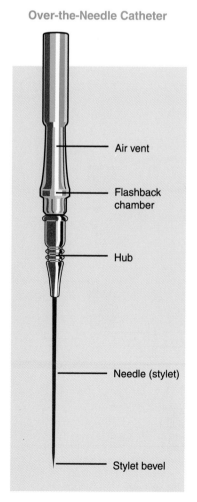

- Air vent
- Flashback chamber
- Hub
- Needle (stylet)
- Stylet bevel

- **Over-the-needle:** This type of catheter is the most common device used for peripheral infusions. The catheter is a hollow tube with a stylet (needle) threaded through the hollow tube that extends beyond the edge of the catheter. The stylet is used to puncture the vein and add rigidity to the catheter for advancing ease into the vein. The catheter has a colored hub that identifies the gauge, a flashback chamber where blood is seen when the vein is accessed, and an air vent that permits the blood to move into the flashback chamber. This type of catheter is an excellent choice with isotonic, normal pH solutions. The Centers for Disease Control and Prevention (CDC) guidelines recommends 96-hour dwell time. Recent research studies have shown that extended dwell times of up to 120 hours have been proven to be safe.

Vein Distention

To complete the selection process, the nurse should identify the available veins that are potential IV sites. To accomplish this task, the vein will need to be distended. The ability of the vein to act as a balloon and enlarge is known as venous distention. To accomplish venous constriction and the resulting distention, the most common method is using a tourniquet. A blood pressure cuff can also be used, which provides a more intense hypoxia of the vein with improved venous distention. This method is especially useful with small veins or the dehydrated patient. Other methods include tapping the vein lightly, applying warm soaks to the arm for 5 to 10 minutes, and lowering the extremity while opening and closing a fist.

Constricting a vein causes hypoxia in the smooth muscles (tunica media) of the vein. The result of the hypoxia is dilation. Dilation allows the vein to engorge with blood, making it visible, palpable, or both. Factors that limit venous distention are anxiety, dehydration, and shock.

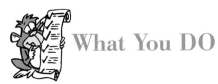

What You DO

Catheter Selection

Selecting the smallest gauge catheter will provide the prescribed flow rate. This choice will maximize hemodilution of the infusate and minimize the trauma of the vein wall by the catheter. When a large-gauge catheter is successfully inserted into a small vein, the catheter/vein ratio is poor, which compromises blood flow and limits hemodilution, leading to vein wall damage. Vein wall damage serves as the major cause of many catheter complications. The greatest chance of vein wall damage is with the small veins in the hand and lower forearm, especially when large catheters are placed.

Because the nurse does not make a final decision about which vein will be selected, it is best to take at least two catheters as a first choice and two catheters in the next smaller gauge. This approach allows some flexibility and limits trips away from the bedside for additional equipment. If using an IV tray or cart, make sure it is stocked with a variety of catheter gauges.

Assess both extremities for bruises, valve location, and areas of pain. Avoid sclerotic (hard) veins; bruised, red, or painful areas; bony prominences; areas of flexion; vein bifurcations and visible valves; and sites below previous venipunctures.

Talk with the patient and determine any preferences and if there is any history with venipuncture successes or failures. Listen to the patient. If the

TAKE HOME POINTS

Factors that limit venous distention are anxiety, dehydration, hypothermia, hypotension, and shock.

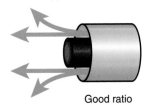

Good ratio

Poor ratio

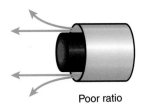

TAKE HOME POINTS

Unrestricted blood flow maximizes hemodilution of drugs and protects the vein wall from damage by the catheter.

Catheter Selection Guide

GAUGE	SELECTION CRITERIA	TIPS
24-26	Used with neonates, pediatric and geriatric patients Suitable for most infusions Excellent choice for very small veins May be used for blood transfusions if thin wall configuration is used	Flow rates may be slower May have slow flashback on insertion Blood bag may need to be divided into two bags to prevent blood infusion hanging too long
22	Appropriate for all infusions including blood transfusion	Not appropriate when high flow rates are required.
20	Minor surgery Cardiac monitoring	Poor selection if patient's veins are too small
18	Surgery Trauma Emergency When high flow rates are required	Not appropriate for small veins of the hands; use largest vein possible; if only small veins are available, consider using central venous access
14-16	Major surgery When high flow rates are required	Increased potential for complications, especially phlebitis if left in place longer than 24 hours; avoid use of larger catheters in small veins, such as the hands; use in large veins only

TAKE HOME POINTS

- The smallest gauge catheter that provides the prescribed flow rate is the best choice.
- Packed red blood cells can be safely administered through 22-gauge catheters and thin wall 24-gauge catheters.
- Both 22-gauge and 24-gauge catheters are sufficient for 75% of all infusions.
- The smallest gauge catheter in the largest vein provides the greatest hemodilution and minimizes vein wall damage.

patient says, for example, "I know this looks like a good vein, but no one has ever successfully stuck it" then do not use the site.

Tourniquet Application

The tourniquet should be applied 4 to 6 inches above the potential insertion site. If a potential insertion site is unknown, then apply the tourniquet on the upper arm. When applying a tourniquet, place it smoothly around the arm, and cross the ends. Stretch the end that is located on top of the cross, and tuck it under. This knot is known as a quick-release knot. Do not pinch the skin. The tourniquet should be tight enough to promote venous distention but not tight enough to impede arterial blood flow. Check for the presence of a radial pulse; it should be present. If the radial pulse is absent, the tourniquet is too

TAKE HOME POINTS

- Do not leave a tourniquet in place longer than 2 minutes.
- Pumping a blood pressure cuff up to just above the diastolic pressure provides excellent venous distention.
- Prolonged distention can cause veins to flatten.
- Over-distention can result in hematoma at the insertion site.

TAKE HOME POINTS

- The area close to the wrist should be avoided for routine venipuncture because of the potential for nerve damage.
- Identify mobility restrictions.

For patients with dark skin, wipe the potential site with an alcohol swab, which will make the potential veins more visible.

Veins that are large and distended in the older adult lack elasticity and are poor sites to use for venipuncture.

tight. If using a blood pressure cuff, inflate to just above the diastolic pressure. If venous distention does not occur, increase pressure just above systolic pressure for up to 1 minute, and then deflate to just above the diastolic pressure.

For the edematous patient, elevate the patient's arm and then tightly wrap a 4-inch Ace bandage, starting at the hand and working up the arm. Leave in place for 3 minutes, and then remove. This technique will temporarily displace some of the fluid. Another method is to apply firm pressure with two or three fingers over the area where a vein should be located. This pressure should visualize the vein and is applied after putting on the tourniquet.

Patients with minimal subcutaneous fat, fragile skin, fragile veins, or those who have altered coagulation require special care. When using a tourniquet, apply loosely over clothing to prevent damage to the skin or bruising. Using the hand to compress the arm may be sufficient to achieve venous distention. If the vein is over-distended, the vein may rupture, causing a hematoma at the insertion site when punctured.

No matter what method for distention is used, the tourniquet should not be left in place longer than 2 minutes. With prolonged distention, the vein wall will relax, and the vein will become flat.

Vein Selection

When the veins are distended, use an index finger to lightly palpate potential veins for venipuncture. Choose veins that are soft and supple. The veins should not pulsate. Start the selection process at the lowest point on the arm. Avoid:

- Bifurcations
- Valves
- Bony prominences
- Areas of flexion
- Arms with loss of motor or sensory function
- Arms with arteriovenous fistula
- The side affected by a CVA or mastectomy

After locating the insertion site, release the tourniquet while preparing the venipuncture equipment and prepare the site. Reapply the tourniquet just before insertion.

If changing from the current site to a new location (restart), use the alternate arm if possible. If this course is not possible, then choose a site at least 3 inches from the previous venipuncture location. The antecubital fossa should be used as a last resort, during an emergency, or for surgery. Large-gauge catheters placed in the antecubital fossa during surgery should be changed within 24 hours to a different site (if patient status permits) to minimize complication potential. If the antecubital vein becomes phlebitic or infiltrates, veins in the forearm below the antecubital site cannot be used until the antecubital area returns to normal.

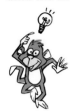

Do You UNDERSTAND?

DIRECTIONS: **Match the items in Column A with the descriptions in Column B.**

Column A

1. _____ Tunica intima
2. _____ Tunica media
3. _____ Tunica adventitia
4. _____ Valves
5. _____ Basilic vein

Column B

a. Responds to a tourniquet with vein distention
b. Location makes venipuncture more difficult
c. Initiates inflammatory response
d. Outer layer is made up of connective tissue
e. Is visible as bulges

DIRECTIONS: **Identify the following statements as *true* (T) or *false* (F).**

6. _____ Veins increase in size with increasing proximity to the heart.
7. _____ It is best to choose a vein located on the affected CVA arm.

DIRECTIONS: **Fill in the blank with the appropriate responses.**

8. Damage to the endothelial cell lining of a vein wall initiates the body to produce an _____ response.

9. Changes in blood volumes occur because the venous system is able to _____ to accommodate increased volume.

10. To avoid vein wall damage, is it better to have a catheter placed in a _____ vein?

11. Two catheter characteristics that affect flow rate are _____ and _____.

Answers: 1. c; 2. a; 3. d; 4. e; 5. b; 6. T; 7. F; 8. inflammatory; 9. expand; 10. larger; 11. internal diameter, length.

DIRECTIONS: **Find the word(s)** *(forward, backward, or scrambled)* **within each line in this puzzle of letters to complete statements 12 to 16.**

```
X V M D E T A R D Y H E D G P
E L B A P L A P B H U O T C E
Q L D U B V T A H Y P O X I A
S S K A O S M K L R N Z I W A
I F A N X I E T Y C V U K S D
C V T Q S H O C K N J R S B N
```

12. Use of a blood pressure cuff enhances distention of small veins in _____ patients.

13. Successful vein engorgement makes a vein _____.

14. _____ of the muscle promotes venous distention.

15. Warm _____ apply to the skin enhance venous distention.

16. Factors that inhibit venous distension are exhibited in patients in the states of _____ and _____.

DIRECTIONS: **Answer the following question.**

17. In which direction would the nurse wrap an edematous arm with an ace bandage to displace the fluid so that a potential IV site can be visualized?

_____

DIRECTIONS: **Fill in the blank with the appropriate response.**

18. To determine that impeded venous flow but not arterial flow has occurred, the nurse should assess for the presence of a _____ _____ when applying a tourniquet to the arm.

What IS Local Anesthesia?

Pain is the leading complication of peripheral IV insertion and is the most common complaint of hospitalized patients. Local anesthesia has been thoroughly documented as an easy, safe, and effective means of reducing the painful adverse effects of peripheral IV cannulation.

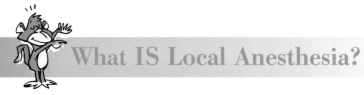

What You NEED TO KNOW

Local anesthesia refers to the topical or intradermal application or administration of drugs to block nerve conduction of painful stimuli within a small, confined area of the body.

Topical local anesthesia: The easiest method of preventing pain from IV insertion is to apply a layer of local anesthetic drugs directly over the vein site. Many special products of such local anesthetics have been developed with the two most common being eutectic mixture of local anesthetics (EMLA) and ELA-max. EMLA and ELA-max are excellent, easy, and convenient ways to minimize the pain of IV cannulation in nonemergency situations. Circumstances such as planned IV catheterization for new patient admissions, for pediatric patients or patients with low pain thresholds, for routine catheter replacements during extended hospitalizations are ideal clinical situations for EMLA and ELA-max use.

- **EMLA:** A eutectic mixture is a mixture of two or more substances that, as a result of being mixed, demonstrates a melting point lower than that of any of its components. EMLA is a nonsterile preparation of 2.5% lidocaine and 2.5% prilocaine that are emulsified in water and thickened into a cream that becomes oily at room temperature or when applied to the skin. Absorption of EMLA is site-specific, being more effective on thin epidermal areas than it is on thick epidermal areas. EMLA is capable of anesthetizing to a maximal depth of 5 to 6 mm below the skin. The duration of the anesthetic effect of EMLA after removal of a 1-hour application is approximately 85 minutes, thus there is no need to rush the catheterization procedure.

- **ELA-max:** The application of ELA-max is essentially the same as that for EMLA. The major difference between the two creams is that ELA-max is composed of 4% lidocaine mixed in a special liposome-encapsulated deliv-

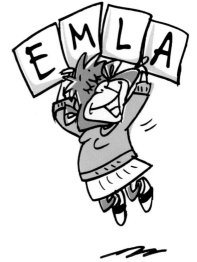

EMLA is *not* recommended for patients under 3 months of age, for patients with known hypersensitivity to lidocaine or prilocaine (extremely rare), or for use on open areas of the skin.

ery system that promotes greater numbness (anesthetizing) in the area to which it is applied.

Intradermal local anesthesia: For situations that will not allow prolonged application time required for the topical creams, an intradermal local anesthetic technique is suitable. An intradermal injection simply refers to the injection or infiltration of medication around the potential site of IV insertion. This technique allows for safe, effective, economical, and rapid local anesthesia immediately preceding IV placement. The only contraindications to local anesthesia for IV catheter placement are the same contraindications for IV catheterization and hypersensitivity to the anesthetic agent.

All local anesthetics can be administered by intradermal injection; however, lidocaine is by far the most commonly used. Lidocaine comes in many different concentrations, and some preparations have a small amount of epinephrine added. For intradermal injection, use the 0.5%, 1%, or 2% concentrations **without** epinephrine. Additionally, the preservative benzyl alcohol is an extremely effective local anesthetic. Benzyl alcohol is the preservative found in some multidose vials of 0.9% normal saline. This flush solution is readily available. If lidocaine is not available, the bacteriostatic saline flush that has benzyl alcohol in it can be used.

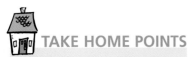

What You DO

Topical analgesics: EMLA should be applied only to intact dermal areas directly over the selected sites of potential venipuncture. EMLA is supplied in a small 5-gram tube, and the recommended application is 2.5 grams (one half the tube) over a 20- to 24-cm^2 (5-inch) area of skin. Squeeze one half of the contents of the tube onto the site and then cover the site with the bio-occlusive dressing provided with the EMLA. (Tegaderm, 3M, or any other occlusive dressing will also work.) Do not worry about spreading the cream; just place the dressing over the little mound of cream, and allow it to spread by itself. Do not prepare the skin with alcohol or other skin cleaners because the natural oils of the skin actually help the EMLA cream to work. The anesthetic effectiveness of EMLA has been determined to be application-time dependent, giving maximal analgesia after 1 to 2 hours of application. However, effectiveness has been documented with application time as little as 5 minutes. A recommended minimal application time is 30 minutes. Because EMLA takes at least an hour to be maximally effective, more than one potential IV site should be prepared simultaneously, just in case IV

TAKE HOME POINTS

Intradermal injection for local anesthesia can cause burning for up to 15 minutes after injection.

TAKE HOME POINTS

Do not clean the skin with alcohol before applying topical analgesics, especially with ELA-max. The natural oils of the skin enhance the penetration of the anesthetic.

placement at one site fails. Be sure to wipe off the cream thoroughly and clean the site with an antiseptic before catheterization because the oily residue from EMLA can make securing the IV with tape difficult. ELA-max needs only a 20- to 30-minute application time to produce an adequate level of analgesia; it does not necessarily need an occlusive dressing as does EMLA. However, a dressing can be used to prevent a mess.

Intradermal local anesthesia: The basic goal of intradermal injection is to do one procedure to minimize the level of discomfort of a second, quite painful procedure. If done improperly, the intradermal injection of a local anesthetic itself can be nearly as painful as starting a smaller gauge IV without local anesthesia. Therefore to first minimize the pain from the local intradermal injection, some helpful information is necessary.

Use the smallest sized needle available for the intradermal injection. Usually, a 27-gauge needle is small enough, but 29-gauges or smaller is ideal.

1. Ensure that the local anesthetic is not cold. Warm solutions of local anesthetic at 98.6° F (37° C) are optimal, but have the local anesthetic at least at room temperature.

2. If using lidocaine, buffer 10 ml of it with 1 ml of 1 mEq/ml of sodium bicarbonate. Although this practice is not imperative, buffering the lidocaine confers two advantages. First, it significantly lessens the transient stinging associated with acidic lidocaine by increasing its pH to that of the body. Second, it lowers the onset time of the lidocaine providing more rapid analgesia. Sodium bicarbonate can be conveniently obtained in 50-ml multidose vials from the hospital pharmacy.

3. Use only a small amount of local anesthetic. Usually, 0.1 to 0.3 ml is enough to provide adequate analgesia.

The technique of local intradermal injection is similar to giving any intradermal injection (e.g., Mantoux test for tuberculosis). Prepare the site with alcohol as usual, and at the selected IV site, insert the anesthetic needle with the bevel upward. Make the approach of the needle at a shallow angle (approximately 5 degrees) to the skin. The needle need not be inserted much farther than the bevel.

The anesthetic needle can be inserted intradermally at the IV site directly on top of the vein if desired. If this method is chosen, gently aspirate to ensure that the needle is not in a vein. An alternative method is to displace the skin over the vein IV site laterally, perform the intradermal injection, and then release the skin back over the vein. This method significantly reduces the chance of venipuncture while making the skin wheal, especially if the patient moves slightly. If performed correctly, the wheal should be about the size of a dime, depending on the amount of anesthetic injected.

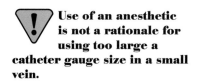

If applying ELA-max on children weighing less than 10 kg (22 lb), be sure that the application area does not exceed 100 cm² (15.5 square inches or approximately 3.9 × 3.9 inches).

Use of an anesthetic is not a rationale for using too large a catheter gauge size in a small vein.

> ⚠ **Use of any anesthetic decreases the patient's ability to recognize pain as a sign of infiltration until the anesthetic wears off.**

Allow at least 15 seconds for the anesthetic to work. If the skin wheal seems to obscure the IV site, gently compress the wheal, and allow the anesthetic to diffuse into the interstitium of the skin. The IV catheter can then be inserted through the same puncture site or anywhere over the wheal and the IV started in the appropriate fashion as described under "Insertion Procedure."

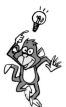

Do You UNDERSTAND?

DIRECTIONS: **Select the best answer to complete each of the following statements.**

1. _____ Topical and intradermal techniques of anesthesia are similar in that they:
   a. Can be used for identical situations when patients need IVs
   b. Attempt to block painful nerve conduction before starting IVs
   c. Require extensive training to be used effectively
   d. Have a large number of side effects

2. _____ When applying topical anesthetics before starting IVs, important considerations include all of the following *except*:
   a. More than one potential IV site should be treated in case one fails.
   b. Analgesic level depends on the dose applied and the length of application time.
   c. Once the topical anesthetic is removed, the nurse should work quickly to start the IV.
   d. Additional care must be taken to ensure safe applications on small children.

3. _____ The mild discomfort from the intradermal injection of local anesthetics can be reduced by all of the following *except*:
   a. Buffering the anesthetic with sodium bicarbonate
   b. Warming the anesthetic
   c. Using very small gauge needles
   d. Injecting the anesthetic at a 45-degree needle angle

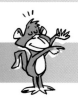

What IS the Insertion Procedure?

The ability to assess, plan, and implement the starting of an IV is what encompasses the insertion procedure. A positive approach to venipuncture, plus an understanding of the procedure and technical practice, will ensure a high percentage of successful venipunctures. Proper handling of the equipment, maintaining aseptic technique, following universal precautions, and preparing the skin before insertion minimize cross-contamination, site infection, and sepsis.

What You NEED TO KNOW

An understanding of skin anatomy and how to use various skin-cleaning preparations is important to enhance infection control. Improper skin preparation can lead to catheter-related infections that result in negative outcomes for the patient. The skin, or the integument, is the largest organ of the body and functions in the areas of support, protection, temperature regulation, and fluid regulation. The skin is composed of two layers: epidermis and dermis.

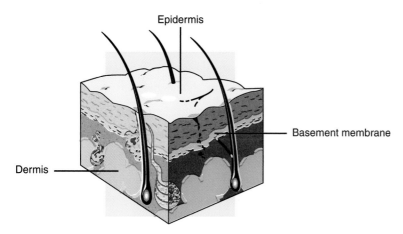

Epidermis

Basement membrane

Dermis

- *Epidermis:* Epidermis is the outermost layer. Thickness varies, with the palms of the hands and the soles of the feet being the thickest and the inner aspect of the forearms being the thinnest area. The epidermis is five layers thick, detects antigens (contact dermatitis), and causes pigmentation. Bacteria are distributed evenly throughout the epidermis layers. Between the epidermis and the dermis is the basement membrane, which adds additional support and flexibility and anchors the epidermis to the dermis. Antigen-antibody response begins here.

- *Dermis:* Dermis is the true skin and is the thickest layer. Sebaceous glands, sweat glands, blood vessels, hair follicles, and nerves are located in the dermis. The dermis is highly sensitive and vascular. The nerves in this layer react to temperature, touch, pressure, and pain. Veins are low-pressure, high-volume reservoirs; they are also able to expand to accommodate increased volume.

It is impossible to sterilize the skin. Interestingly, 80% of the transient and resident microflora live in the first five layers of the epidermis (epidermis consists of approximately 25 layers in a space of 1 mm). Bacteria will repopulate the surface within 3 hours. Common skin preparations are alcohol, iodophor, chlorhexidine, and "one-step" preparations.

- *Alcohol:* Alcohol is the minimum skin cleanser. The most common concentration for skin preparation is 70%.
  Advantages: Rapid effect and greatest reduction of bacteria counts
  Disadvantages: Dries the skin, only effective on clean skin and when wet; dries the skin

- *Iodophor (povidone-iodine):* Iodophor must be in contact with the skin for at least 2 minutes for the bound iodine to become active. With drying, the bacteriocidal activity declines.
  Advantages: Water soluble, less irritating than iodine, nonstaining
  Disadvantages: Prolonged contact time required; rinsing removes bacteriocidal effects, deactivated by organic material such as blood, and can be contaminated

- *Chlorhexidine* (ChloraPrep formulation of 2% chlorhexidine in 70% isopropyl alcohol).
  Advantages: Active for 5 to 6 hours; with repeated use, effect increases (persistence); not inactivated by organic material, toxicity uncommon, not absorbed
  Disadvantages: pH dependent; neutralized by hard tap water, nonionic surfactants, and soap

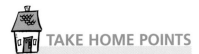

TAKE HOME POINTS

If the person is allergic to iodine or seafood, the use of iodophor products is contraindicated.

Some one-step preparations dry shiny, and the glare from lighting can make vein visualization difficult.

- *One-step:* Combination preparations that contain alcohol, povidone iodine or other approved germicide, and skin protectants that permit cleaning the skin in one step (e.g., Persist (Becton Dickinson, Salt Lake City, Utah), IV Prep (Smith & Nephew, Largo, Fla.).

Handwashing prevents cross-contamination between patients and nurses. The objective of handwashing is to remove resident skin flora. Even though handwashing is recommended 100% of the time, the actual practice occurs only 50% of the time. The duration is shorter than is recommended. After wetting hands thoroughly, use a vigorous scrubbing action for 10 to 15 seconds with 3 to 5 ml of antimicrobial soap (remember thumbs, nail beds, and rings). Thorough coverage and friction on all surfaces of the hands are required. Thoroughly rinse hands, and use a paper towel to turn off the faucet.

A moisture-proof barrier should be placed under the arm to prevent contamination of the bed linen or furniture during venipuncture procedure. The Occupational Safety and Health Administration (OSHA) guidelines require the use of needle-protector systems and needle-free access systems. All sharps should be placed in a needle-protected container.

Be aware that many patients are afraid of venipuncture. Anxiety can result in a systemic vasomotor response known as vagal reaction. Although usually benign and self-limiting, the symptoms of anxiety can include:

- Fall in systolic blood pressure
- Sinus bradycardia
- Pallor and cold sweating
- Nausea
- Dizziness
- Fainting
- Venous spasm

What You DO

Collect the needed equipment: tourniquet, skin preparations, tape, gauze, moisture-proof barrier, dressing, and four catheters (two different gauges—the selected one and the next smaller gauge). Patient identification is confirmed, and introductions are made. Review the procedure with the patient and answer any questions. The explanation should include the purpose of the therapy, duration of the therapy, the type of therapy (continuous, intermittent, IV push), any restrictions to activity, and signs and symptoms that should be reported to the nurse.

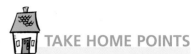

TAKE HOME POINTS

Aqueous benzalkonium-like solutions and hexachlorophene are not to be used as IV skin preparations.

TAKE HOME POINTS

- Artificial nails can harbor fungus and bacteria and should not be worn during patient care.
- Gloves must be worn whenever the potential exists for contact with blood, body fluids, excretions, and contaminated surfaces.
- Change gloves with each new patient contact.

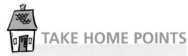

TAKE HOME POINTS

Patients have the right to refuse venipuncture. To force a patient is legally considered assault and battery.

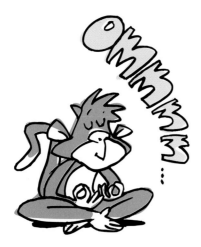

Do not touch the skin once it has been prepared. If the skin must be palpated again, then the skin should be prepared again.

TAKE HOME POINTS

Vein stabilization is critical to successful venipuncture.

TAKE HOME POINTS

If the nurse has trouble with veins rupturing (blowing), he or she should lower the angle of insertion. The high angle is allowing the catheter to puncture the back wall of the vein instead of advancing up the vein.

A calm, confident demeanor can reduce patient anxiety. Wash hands, then apply gloves. Venipuncture can be performed while sitting or standing. The patient and nurse should be comfortable. There should be adequate light, a place for all of the equipment that is easily reachable, and a sharps container for the stylet once it is removed from the catheter.

Clean site: Clean a 3- to 4-inch area around the proposed venipuncture site. Use friction. If using alcohol and iodophor, clean first with the alcohol and then with the iodophor. An easy method involves using a circular motion starting at the venipuncture site and working outward. This action prevents recontamination of the potential insertion site. Allow alcohol to air dry completely before preparing with the iodophor. Do not fan, blow on, or blot the area. Skin prepared bacteriocidal activity occurs while wet. Quick drying minimizes bacteriocidal action. Using alcohol to remove the iodophor for better visualization negates the antimicrobial action of the iodophor. If using chlorhexidine or combination preparations, clean the area using the same circular motion for 30 to 45 seconds, and allow to dry completely.

Catheter use: Open up the catheter and remove the protector. Be careful not to touch the catheter. Inspect the catheter for irregularities such as a bur (rough spot). If any irregularities are present, discard and use a new catheter. With some peripheral catheters, it is necessary to rotate the catheter around the stylet to loosen the connection. There are numerous needle-protective systems available. These catheters are designed to protect the stylet tip when it is removed from the catheter. Know the manufacturer's guidelines for preparing the catheter for venipuncture and activating the needle protective system. Grasp the cannula behind the hub with the bevel up.

To be successful with **venipuncture,** there are seven steps to follow.

- *Step 1:* Stabilize the vein by placing a thumb on the vein below the insertion site and pulling down away from the site. The skin should be taut. The vein will appear to flatten somewhat, but it remains engorged below the skin. Tight skin is easier to pierce than is loose skin. If the skin wrinkles in an attempt to enter the vein, the skin is not tight enough.
- *Step 2:* Angle of entry is important. Keep the angle as low as possible so that when vein entry is accomplished, the catheter tip is in the vein (15 degrees for superficial veins and slightly higher for deeper veins). Keep the thumb out of the insertion path. When inserting over the thumb, the insertion angle will be too steep, and the catheter will pass through the back wall of the vein. When the angle is too low, the catheter will not penetrate the vein.
- *Step 3:* Holding the flashback chamber (do not hold the hub), with stylet bevel up and the catheter pointing in the direction of blood flow,

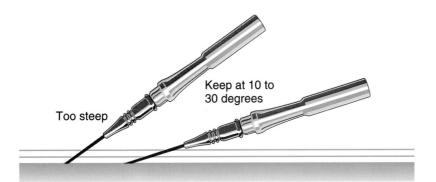

Keep at 10 to
30 degrees

Too steep

pierce the skin directly over the vein. This ensures that the needle will enter the vein. When piercing the vein from the side, the needle pushes the vein away as it attempts to pierce it. Enter the skin and the vein in one motion. Do not go through the skin and then the vein. Insert at least $^1/4$ inch of the catheter. This length ensures both the stylet tip and the catheter are inside the vein.

- **Step 4:** When blood is observed in the flashback chamber, lower the catheter almost to the skin level, and pull back on the stylet slightly to "hood" (hide) the needle tip in the catheter. While holding onto the hub (colored area), slide the catheter and the stylet forward into the vein. Do not touch the end of the hub. This action will contaminate the catheter. If the cannula is pushed off from the stylet, the catheter loses the stiffening that the stylet adds, which may make advancing the catheter difficult. If the catheter will not advance, the most common reason is the catheter is not in the vein (only the stylet tip punctured the vein). Once the catheter has been completely advanced into the vein, release the tourniquet. Remember, early tourniquet release may cause the vein to go flat, inhibiting catheter advancement.

- **Step 5:** While holding the catheter hub with the thumb and index finger of the nondominant hand, apply light pressure with the remaining fingers to the vein above the tip of the catheter and remove the stylet. The vein compression minimizes blood flowing from the catheter. With practice, a venipuncture can be bloodless. Discard the stylet in an approved sharps container.

- **Step 6:** Attach a cap and flush with saline (**not** heparin lock solution) to check patency (for intermittent use), or attach the primed extension set or primary administration set (for continuous use). Lower the IV container below the level of the heart. Blood flow into the tubing confirms successful catheter placement. If blood flashback is present, but the IV solution flow rate is sluggish, the tip of the catheter may be up

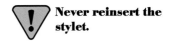
Never reinsert the stylet.

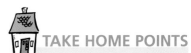
TAKE HOME POINTS

With extreme dehydration or hypovolemia, there can be an absence of a blood flashback.

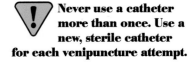
Never use a catheter more than once. Use a new, sterile catheter for each venipuncture attempt.

against the wall of the vein, and repositioning of the catheter may be necessary. If the site swells, feels cool to touch, or both, stop the infusion or flushing. This condition indicates infiltration and an unsuccessful attempt.

- *Step 7*: Secure the catheter to minimize catheter movement. Several methods are commonly used to secure catheters, including the Chevron method, the H method, and the U method. Use the taping method that best secures the catheter. Sterile tape should be applied to the catheter if required. Remember, tearing the tape before venipuncture and attaching the tape to the nonsterile bed rail should not be done. If done, the bed rail will contaminate the tape. Vancomycin-resistant enterococci (VRE) have been found living for 24 hours on bed rails. Visual assessment of the insertion site should not be obstructed by tape.

TAKE HOME POINTS

If the patient is allergic to tape, use nonallergic tape. The tape should not be placed directly over the venipuncture site. Use a taping method that best secures the catheter.

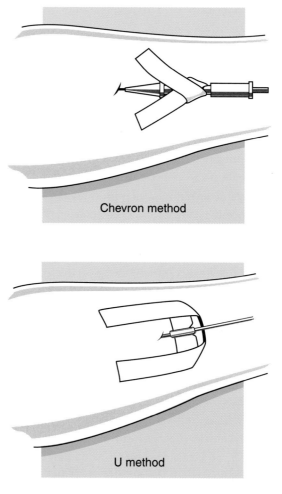

Chevron method

U method

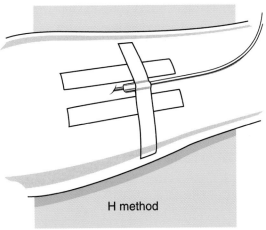

H method

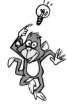

Do You UNDERSTAND?

1. On the first clock, place an "X" on the hour that signifies the time lapse between cleansing the skin for venipuncture and bacteria repopulating the skin surface.
2. On the second clock, place an "X" on the clock that signifies the number of minutes needed for bound iodine to become active once it is wiped on the skin before venipuncture.

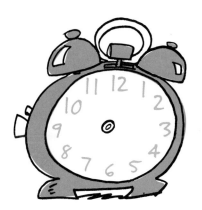
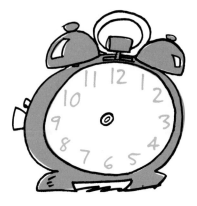

Answers: 1. 3 hours; 2. 2 minutes.

DIRECTIONS: **Provide short answers for the following questions.**

3. What is the most effective nursing intervention to prevent cross-contamination between patients and nurses?

_____

4. The use of the term "flashback" during insertion of an IV means what has occurred?

_____

5. If a flashback has occurred, but the nurse is unable to thread the catheter what might be the cause?

_____.

6. Where should the stylet be discarded?

_____

What IS Applying the Dressing?

The function of placing a dressing over the insertion site is to protect the insertion site from trauma while keeping the site dry and clean. Catheter movement can cause vein wall damage and insertion site trauma.

What You NEED TO KNOW

Infusion Nursing Society (INS) standards of infusion nursing practice state that the catheter should be stabilized so as not to interfere with visual site assessment or impede the delivery of the prescribed flow rate. Transparent dressings or tape and gauze are commonly used for peripheral IV site dressings.

- *Transparent or semipermeable membrane dressings*

  Advantages: Insertion site visible, flexible, comfortable; provides a barrier (moisture, bacterial, and viral); CDC recommends use; comes in a variety of sizes and designs

  Disadvantages: Inhibits (degree varies with dressing) moisture vapor transmission from the skin, easily pulled off; excessive diaphoresis can cause loss of adhesion; may not provide adequate stabilization

- *Tape and gauze dressing*

    Advantages: Provides moisture vapor transmission, absorbs moisture, inexpensive

    Disadvantages: Lack of insertion site visibility; daily change required; not a moisture, bacterial, or viral barrier

What You DO

Dressings are applied at the time of venipuncture and are changed when loose, wet, or no longer intact; at the time of routine change; or daily, if tape and gauze are used. Aseptic technique should be maintained throughout the procedure. Applying a skin protector before dressing application enhances dressing adhesion and protects the skin. Skin protectors should be allowed to dry completely before the dressing is applied.

A catheter protection device, such as a plastic dome (e.g., IV house [see color plate 1]) or a securement device (e.g., StatLock [see color plate 2]), can be used to enhance catheter stabilization and insertion site protection.

When using a transparent dressing, it should not be placed over the hub connection. If the hub connection is covered, changing the tubing or caps is difficult. Transparent dressings should be secured around the catheter hub and compressed to the skin to provide an occlusive seal. Additional tape can be added to ensure this occlusive seal. The tubing attached to the IV catheter should be taped with a stress-prevention loop, limiting direct pulling on the catheter. Once the dressing application is complete, label the dressing either directly on the dressing with ballpoint pen or using an adhesive label with the date, time, catheter gauge, catheter length, and initials.

Applying a skin protector helps maintain skin integrity in older adults, as well as any patient with fragile skin.

Securement devices are particularly useful with children and confused patients.

Never tape all the way around the arm. Doing so can act as a tourniquet, which increases the risk of infiltration.

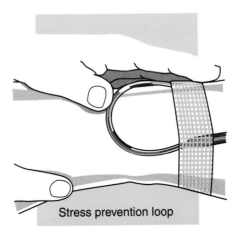

Stress prevention loop

TAKE HOME POINTS

- Always pull the dressing toward the insertion site.
- Dressing changes for peripheral IVs are rarely needed because the IV site is routinely changed every 96 hours, if not before.

Never use scissors to remove tape. The catheter or patient may be inadvertently cut. If tape removal pads are not available, alcohol can help with removal. Apply tension to the dressing as well.

Arm boards are occasionally needed, especially if the only available venipuncture site is in an area of flexion. An arm board should be placed so that it does not cover the insertion site and is secured in a manner that does not impede the infusion or circulation. Arm boards should be removed at established intervals according to institution policy. Restraints should not be applied near the IV site.

When changing a dressing, it is important to stabilize the catheter. It is very easy to pull the catheter out when removing a dressing. Always secure the catheter when removing a dressing. Lift a corner of the dressing, and then (while rubbing the skin with a tape remover pad) pull the dressing up toward the insertion site. This procedure will ensure ease of dressing removal. If the patient has a hairy arm, then pull the dressing off not only toward the insertion site, but also in the direction that the hair grows, which minimizes pulling out the hair.

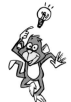

Do You UNDERSTAND?

DIRECTIONS: **Match the equipment to it usage.**

Equipment

1. _____ Dome
2. _____ Arm board
3. _____ Gauze
4. _____ Tape

Usage

a. Is used over area of flexion
b. Is a catheter protection device
c. Absorbs moisture
d. Is used as an occlusive sealing agent

DIRECTIONS: **Write the answer to the following question in the space provided.**

5. Why does the nurse never secure an IV by taping completely around and encircling the arm?

_____

_____

Answers: 1. b; 2. a; 3. c; 4. d; 5. increases chance of infiltration.

What IS a Flushing Procedure?

The flushing procedure is a treatment designed to rid the catheter of whatever is in the device, a treatment designed to maintain patency of the catheter for future use, or both. The flushing procedure should always be done carefully and with minimal force applied to the syringe plunger. Veins and catheters have different elastic capabilities. All patients and all catheters are not the same. There are no universal standards available to guide syringe choice for flushing.

What You NEED TO KNOW

When applying force with the thumb on a syringe plunger, pressure is exerted on the catheter and vein. The same amount of force applied to smaller syringes results in higher pressure.

$$\text{Pressure} = \frac{\text{force applied}}{\text{area}}$$

What You DO

It is important to become familiar with how a patient's IV catheter feels during flushing to detect changes. The saline–administer medication– saline (SAS) method should always be used.

- *Saline:* First use saline to remove any heparin or other medications present in the tubing to prevent any incompatibility between heparin and the medication and to check for catheter patency and vein integrity. Slowly flush the catheter while palpating above the catheter tip for signs of cool skin temperature and swelling. If the patient complains of pain during flushing, stop. Pain may be the first sign of a problem. Reposition the arm and flush again slowly. If pain persists, the safest intervention is to dis-

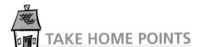

TAKE HOME POINTS

Using the same force, a smaller syringe will exert more pressure on a vein, thereby increasing the chance of infiltration.

continue use of the IV site and relocate the IV. If resistance is felt, stop flushing. Additional force should be avoided. Assess the dressing and tape for constrictions. The dressing may need to be removed to check the insertion site. Catheters can become kinked at the insertion site. Never reinsert a catheter that has tracked back out of the insertion site and kinked. If possible, retape and redress the catheter and flush again. If this is not possible, the catheter will need to be discontinued and restarted in a new location.

- *Administer medication or additive:* After the catheter has been flushed smoothly, without resistance and without any signs of problems, administer the medication.
- *Saline:* After the medication has been infused, flush the catheter with saline again to clear the line of any residual medication and to move the medication into the main circulation. Medication left in small peripheral veins can cause irritation. Final flushing of peripheral catheters with heparinized saline does not affect occlusion rates and is not cost effective. However, follow the institution's protocol. If heparinized saline is used, it is commonly a 10-unit concentration and 1 cc volume. Maintain positive pressure during and when completing the flush to prevent reflux of blood into the catheter tip. To establish positive pressure with nonpositive pressure caps, clamp the line while flushing or maintain forward push on the plunger as the syringe is removed from the access. With positive pressure caps, disconnect the syringe first and then close the extension set clamp.

TAKE HOME POINTS

If flushing through a Y site, use the one closest to the catheter insertion site. Remember to pinch off the tubing just above the Y site with the fingers, then flush and release the pinch-off.

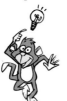

Do You UNDERSTAND?

DIRECTIONS: **Fill in the blanks in the following sentences using the words pressure, saline, pain, and resistance.**

1. The "S" in the SAS method of flushing stands for _____.

2. If the nurse is flushing a peripheral IV and feels _____, flushing should be stopped.

Answers: 1. saline; 2. resistance.

3. _____ equals the force applied divided by the area.

4. _____ is a sign of phlebitis.

DIRECTIONS: **Answer the following questions.**

5. When flushing an IV catheter, should it be done fast or slow?

   _____

6. The nurse is flushing an IV and meets resistance. The arm is repositioned, and flushing is attempted once again. A small amount of swelling is noticed just above the IV insertion site. What should be done next?

   _____

   _____

   _____

What IS the Removal Procedure?

Removal procedures are the means whereby the peripheral IV medication is discontinued (temporarily or permanently) and the IV catheter is taken out of the vein.

What You NEED TO KNOW

Catheters are removed at the completion of therapy, when any sign or symptom of a complication occurs, or when the catheter has been in place for 96 hours.

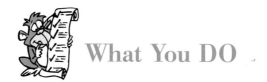

What You DO

First, apply gloves because of the potential exposure to blood. To remove a catheter, first remove the tape and dressing. Remove tape carefully by pulling in the direction of hair growth. The use of adhesive solvents or alcohol can dissolve the adhesive. While holding the catheter with the nondominant hand, loosen the edge of the transparent dressing with the dominant hand. Stretch the dressing a little at a time. This technique will release the dressing from the skin. Work toward the insertion site. Apply the adhesive remover or alcohol under the remaining dressing as it is stretched. This procedure can be time consuming but will minimize patient discomfort. Once the dressing and all tape have been removed, pull the catheter out parallel to the skin. Immediately cover the site with a dry gauze pad. Do **not** use an alcohol pad. Alcohol will burn and prolong bleeding. Elevate the extremity and hold pressure until the bleeding has stopped (3 to 5 minutes). If the patient has any reason for increased bleeding time, pressure will have to be applied for a longer period. Tape the gauze in place, if necessary.

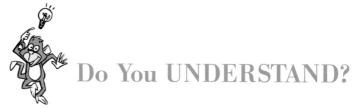

Do You UNDERSTAND?

DIRECTIONS: **Place a check mark next to the statements that signifies when a peripheral IV catheter should be removed.**

1. _____ Catheter has been in place for 96 hours.
2. _____ Heparin lock has been in place for 24 hours.
3. _____ There is no longer a need for IV access.
4. _____ The critically ill patient has no other noticeable venous access on assessment.

DIRECTIONS: **Place the number "1" next to the first intervention, the number "2" next to the second intervention, and so on until number "6" indicating the correct order in removing a peripheral IV catheter.**

5. _____ Hold pressure on IV site until bleeding stops.

6. _____ Pull catheter out parallel to the skin.

7. _____ Apply dry gauze to IV site.

8. _____ Remove tape from IV site.

9. _____ Remove IV dressing.

10. _____ Elevate the extremity.

DIRECTIONS: **Provide two reasons why an alcohol pad should never be used on an IV site that just had an IV removed.**

11. _____

_____

What IS Documentation?

Documentation is a legal, ethical, and professional responsibility. After the insertion procedure is complete, the nurse must document the patient's record. Documentation outlines the care the nurse has provided and the patient's response.

What You NEED TO KNOW

Documentation of a peripheral IV is the legal application of charting the care the nurse has given the patient in relation to their peripheral IV therapy.

What You DO

After the insertion procedure is complete, it must be documented in the patient's record. The documentation should include:

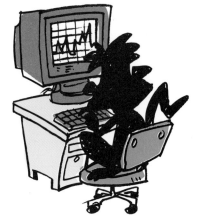

- Date and time of procedure
- Arm (right or left)
- Location on the arm (upper, mid, or lower)
- Vein name
- Catheter (gauge and length)
- Infusion (type, rate, and presence of an electronic infusion device)
- Unsuccessful attempts
- Condition of the site before and after procedure
- Patient comments
- Use of arm board or refusal, if appropriate
- Patient tolerance of procedure
- Instructions given to patient and family
- Interventions resulting from complications (e.g., cold or warm pack applied to IV area)
- Nurse's signature and title, once entry is complete

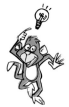

Do You UNDERSTAND?

DIRECTIONS: **Place a check next to the best answer to each of the following questions.**

1. Who has the responsibility of documenting the insertion procedure of a peripheral IV?

   a. _____ Secretary

   b. _____ Nurse manager

   c. _____ Person who inserted the IV

   d. _____ Any registered nurse assigned to the patient

2. Mrs. Woo, a 28-year-old ambulatory postoperative thyroidectomy patient, has had a peripheral IV in her left cephalic vein for the last 96 hours. Where would the assessment occur to restart her peripheral IV?

a. _____ Left jugular   c. _____ Left arm
b. _____ Right groin   d. _____ Right arm

What IS Patient Education?

An educated patient is one who is fully informed and therefore able to actively participate in his or her care. This interaction will enhance successful outcomes. Patients have the human and legal right to receive information on all aspects of their care.

What You NEED TO KNOW

The patient must understand the following:
- Mobility restrictions
- Signs and symptoms of problems that must be reported
- Care and maintenance of the catheter, the dressing, and the IV administration equipment
- All procedures required for successful IV delivery
- When medical assistance is necessary
- How to call for help

If the patient is unable to understand this information, then educate the patient's caregiver. Patient's readiness to learn varies. Written material is helpful. The nurse may have to read the information to the patient before leaving it with him or her.

What You DO

Assess the patient's knowledge level, motivation, ability to cooperate, and readiness to learn. Without motivation and readiness, learning cannot take place.

Answer: 2. d.

Assess barriers that may interfere with the nurse's ability to communicate effectively with the patient, including the following:

- Age
- Cultural barriers
- Language barriers
- Level of education
- Level of anxiety and stress
- Cooperation
- Coherence

Develop a plan of action to minimize barrier impact. For example, use an interpreter if required. Remember: if the patient does not understand the information, the patient teaching is not effective. Set up times for reinforcing education, such as at the time of site assessments. It is important not only to show the patient what to do, but also to have the patient demonstrate what should be done or verbally repeat instructions. Allow time for patient questions.

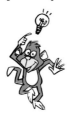

Do You UNDERSTAND?

DIRECTIONS: **Fill in the blanks with the correct answer.**

1. Patients must be educated regarding IV therapy so they can understand:
   a. Restrictions associated with _____.
   b. Signs and _____ of infiltration.
   c. Care and maintenance of the _____, dressing, and equipment.
   d. How to call for _____.

DIRECTIONS: **Identify the following statements as *true* (T) or *false* (F).**

2. Patients may not be ready to learn if they are:
   a. _____ Under extreme stress
   b. _____ Women
   c. _____ Over educated
   d. _____ Not motivated

CHAPTER

3 Peripheral Complications

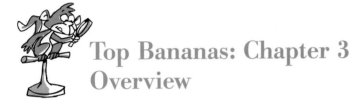

Top Bananas: Chapter 3 Overview

The container, the flow rate, the administration tubing, the dressing, the intravenous (IV) catheter, the insertion site, and patient response are very important for the early detection of problems or complications. Early detection and appropriate intervention are required if the prescribed IV therapy is going to be successfully maintained. It is important to remember that, although not all complications can be eliminated, the best intervention is prevention. The nurse must be knowledgeable about IV solutions, the purpose of the IV solution, and the anticipated action of the solution, as well as any contraindications, side effects, and adverse reactions. Peripheral complications, which occur at or near the insertion site, are the most common complications of IV therapy and are not usually life threatening. Early detection and treatment can prevent more serious complications from occurring.

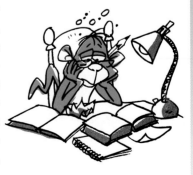

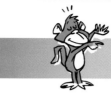

What IS Mechanical Failure?

Mechanical failure occurs when the prescribed flow rate with an infusion is not able to be maintained. It is important to determine if the IV delivery system is functioning properly.

What You NEED TO KNOW

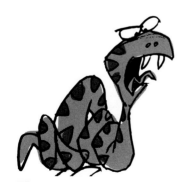

In some electronic infusion devices, alarms can be turned off or "silenced." This practice should not be done in nursing care.

It is important to be familiar with all IV equipment that is being used in the facility. IV equipment is updated and changed often. Understand how to use all electronic infusion devices. Become familiar with the meaning of all alarms. It is the nurse's responsibility to understand the correct procedures for IV administration and appropriate interventions when problems arise.

What You DO

Assess that the solution container has been completely spiked with the appropriate administration set for the container. Make sure that the tubing is hanging straight without any kinks. Assess that the filter is not filled with air and that all clamps are open. Check the dressing and the tape for constriction. Make sure that nothing is causing pressure on the IV catheter or the vein path. Carefully flush the catheter using minimal pressure to identify any resistance. If the administration tubing can be disconnected easily from the catheter, see if the solution flows freely. If the fluid flows freely, then the problem is with the catheter, not the administration set. If the solution does not flow freely, then the problem is with the administration set.

In rare instances, there can be a malfunctioning pump. However, the pump is most likely not broken when the continual occlusion alarm sounds. Rather, there is some other cause for increased resistance in the administration set and catheter.

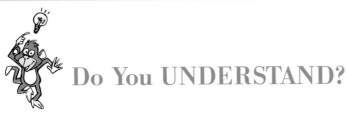

Do You UNDERSTAND?

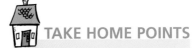
DIRECTIONS: Fill in the blanks with the appropriate response.

1. Early detection of complications from peripheral IV's includes assessing the:

   a. Fluid _____

   b. Flow _____

   c. Administration _____ and _____-_____

   d. _____ catheter

   e. Insertion _____

   f. Patient _____

DIRECTIONS: Place a check next to all the phrases that can cause mechanical failure in a peripheral IV.

2. _____ Tourniquet is left on peripheral IV arm.
3. _____ Infusion has <50 ml left in the dose to be infused.
4. _____ Tubing is kinked.
5. _____ Clamp is in the "open" position on the IV line.

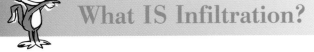

What IS Infiltration?

The Infusion Nursing Society (INS) defines infiltration as the inadvertent administration of a nonvesicant solution or medication into surrounding tissues as a result of dislodgment of a cannula (see color plate 3).

What You NEED TO KNOW

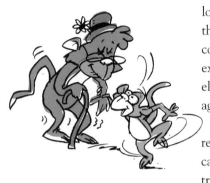

Veins are capable of expanding to hold increased fluid volume. A normal, healthy vessel can withstand 1.9 pounds per inch (psi) before it ruptures. However, many veins in ill patients are more fragile and will rupture at far lower levels of pressure compared with those of healthy individuals. When the vein is overextended, the vein will break, even if the catheter is placed correctly inside the vein. This reason is why in the presence of swelling with existing catheters, a blood return is *not* an indicator of vein integrity. Vein elasticity is especially diminished in older adults. Vein fragility increases with age, poor nutritional status, and long-term steroid usage.

Infiltration may also result when the catheter damages the vein wall as a result of catheter movement. This problem is exacerbated when a large catheter is placed in a small vein. Poor insertion technique can cause infiltration. With high-angle insertion, the potential for the catheter to enter the vein and nick or exit the back wall of the vein is increased.

Causes of infiltration include:
- Inappropriate vein selection
- Poor catheter/vein ratio
- Poor insertion technique
- Poor vein elasticity
- Increased vein fragility
- Use of high pressure (either manually or electronically)
- Over manipulation of the catheter
- Poor dressing management

Signs and symptoms of infiltration include:
- Skin tightness
- Swelling
- Pain, tenderness, discomfort
- Cool skin temperature
- Blanching
- Slowing down of the rate of flow
- Leaking at the site or wet dressing

When infiltration occurs, the infusion rate is compromised; the extremity below the infiltration is lost to future IVs until the infiltration site is resolved; and the patient suffers pain, possibly loss of mobility, and interference with therapy.

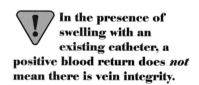 Veins in older adults require decreased levels of pressure to rupture because of a loss of vessel elasticity.

In the presence of swelling with an existing catheter, a positive blood return does *not* mean there is vein integrity.

TAKE HOME POINTS

Edema of the hands, forearms, or both can have different causes other than infiltration, such as immobilization, heart failure, or superior vena cava syndrome.

What You DO

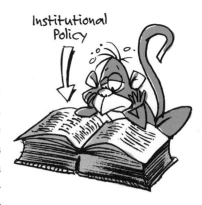

Although all infiltrations cannot be prevented, close site monitoring and communication with the patient may minimize the effects. There are no specific guidelines governing the frequency of monitoring catheter sites by the Joint Commission on Accreditation of Healthcare Organizations (JCAHO) or the INS. Both organizations recommend that institutions set a policy and procedure governing the frequency and method for site inspection. Specific intervals should be established. Commonly, IV sites should be inspected *at least* every 2 hours. In high-risk environments such as pediatric, geriatric, oncology, and critical care units, inspection should be more frequent. The nurse should make it a practice to assess the IV site each time he or she in the patient's room.

Prevention: Preventing infiltration requires implementing actions that minimize the potential for vein wall damage. Actions include:

1. *Minimize vein wall puncture.*
   - The smallest catheter and the largest vein should always be selected.
   - Prominences and areas of flexion should be avoided as potential insertion sites because these sites increase the potential for mechanical damage to the vein by catheter movement.
   - IV dressing should be secured, and catheter movement should be minimized.

2. *Minimize catheter and vein restrictions.*
   - IV catheters should not be placed under restraints. If an IV is placed below a restraint, then the restraint must be applied in such a way as not to constrict the arm.
   - Arm boards should be well padded. Tape that goes over the arm above the insertion site should be double-faced to prevent the tape from adhering to the skin.

3. *Minimize overextension of the vein.*
   - Flush slowly with minimal pressure on the plunger. If resistance is felt, do not overcome this pressure with additional pressure. Stop, reposition the arm, and check the catheter, dressing, and insertion site. Repeated, rapid flushing can over extend the vein repeatedly weakening it.

Assessment: It is important to closely assess the entire area around the patient's insertion site. IV fluid can continue to flow into the tissue of

TAKE HOME POINTS

Frequent monitoring of the infusion site is very important. This practice allows the nurse to identify complications early and institute the appropriate treatment.

Electronic pumps do not recognize infiltration. Electronic pumps will not sound an alarm until the preset pressure limit is reached.

TAKE HOME POINTS

The catheter may be positioned in such a way as to allow a small blood return while the vein wall integrity is compromised, allowing infiltration.

patients with poor tissue turgor (e.g., malnourished patients, older adults) for prolonged periods with no interruption of the flow rate. It is important to lift the patient's arm and observe under the arm. Fluid can collect dependently, and although the area around the insertion site looks normal, the area under the arm can be swollen. Compare both arms in size and shape. An excellent test for infiltration is to lightly compress the vein above the catheter tip using a finger. If the IV solution continues to flow, suspect infiltration. When lightly palpating the skin above the IV catheter tip, the area will feel firm or even hard with infiltration; it will also feel cool.

Treatment: If infiltration is suspected, the IV solution must be stopped and the IV catheter removed. Research has shown that elevating the arm or applying warm compresses does not affect the fluid reabsorption time. The fluid has a different osmolarity than does the tissue. The body's response is to increase fluid in the area to dilute the drug and return the tissue osmolarity to normal. With hypertonic solutions, such as $D_{10}W$ and D_5LR, heat increases the size of the infiltration and slows reabsorption. Therefore apply a cool compress to the infiltrated area. Do not elevate the extremity.

When restarting the IV as a result of infiltration, if possible, use the opposite extremity. If the same extremity must be used, place the IV at least 3 inches above the infiltration site and on the opposite side of the extremity.

Documentation is very important with infiltration. Documentation should include not only the visual assessment, but also the patient's response and interventions instituted. Infiltration is a frequent cause for malpractice claims. The INS has developed an infiltration scale.

Infiltration Scale

GRADE	CRITERIA
0	No symptoms
1	Skin blanched, edema <1 inch, cool to touch, with or without pain
2	Skin blanched, edema 1 to 6 inches, cool to touch, with or without pain
3	Skin blanched, translucent, gross edema >6 inches, cool to touch, mild-to-moderate pain, possible numbness
4	Skin blanched, translucent, skin tight, leaking, skin discolored, bruised, swollen, gross edema >6 inches, deep pitting tissue edema, circulatory
5	Impairment, moderate to severe pain, infiltration of any amount of blood product, irritant or vesicant

TAKE HOME POINTS

Do not apply cool compresses with chemotherapeutic agents with vinca alkaloid infiltrations. Apply heat.

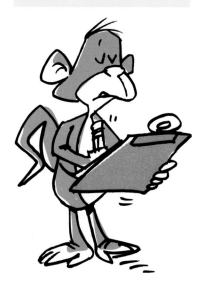

TAKE HOME POINTS

The infiltrated area may have a normal appearance, even though one half of the infiltrated fluid has not been absorbed.

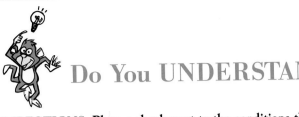

Do You UNDERSTAND?

DIRECTIONS: **Place a check next to the conditions that increase a patients risk of IV infiltration.**

1. _____ Use of steroids for 6 months
2. _____ Protein malnutrition
3. _____ Use of tourniquet during IV insertion procedure
4. _____ Large size IV catheter in a small vein
5. _____ High-pressure electronic pump used to regulate IV flow
6. _____ Patient is between the ages of 18 and 35 years

DIRECTIONS: **Fill in the blanks for signs and symptoms of a peripheral IV infiltration.**

7. Slow rate of _____ of IV

8. _____ dressing of IV site

9. _____ skin temperature

DIRECTIONS: **Fill in the blanks with the appropriate response.**

10. Peripheral IV sites should be assessed at least every _____ hour(s).

DIRECTIONS: **Place a check next to all those that apply.**

11. Inspection of peripheral IVs should be done more often in what high-risk groups or environments?
   a. _____ Adults
   b. _____ Older adults
   c. _____ Patients with cancer
   d. _____ Pediatric patients
   e. _____ Critical care unit
   f. _____ Men

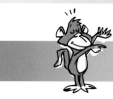

What IS Extravasation?

Extravasation is defined by the INS as the inadvertent administration of a vesicant solution, vesicant medication, or both into surrounding tissue (see color plates 4, 5, 6, and 7).

What You NEED TO KNOW

Vesicants cause tissue death (necrosis) and tissue falling off from the body (sloughing).

Vesicant Drugs

MEDICATION	CLASSIFICATION	USES
Amphotericin B	Antifungal	Histoplasmosis, mucosis, aspergillosis, candidiasis, septicemia, meningitis
Calcium gluconate	Electrolyte replacement	Treatment of hypocalcemia, hypermagnesemia, hypoparathyroidism, hyperphosphatemia, vitamin D deficiency, cardiac toxicity caused by hyperkalemia
Caunorubicin	Antineoplastic	Cancer
Contrast media	Radiography enhancer	Computed tomographic scans, gallium scans, radiologic scans
Dacarbazine	Antineoplastic	Cancer
Dactinomycin	Antineoplastic	Cancer
Daunorubicin	Antineoplastic	Cancer
Docetaxel (Taxotere)	Antineoplastic	Cancer
Dopamine	Adrenergic, catecholamine	Shock, increase perfusion, hypotension
Doxorubicin	Antineoplastic	Cancer
High concentration potassium chloride	Electrolyte replacement	Hypokalemia
Idarubicin	Antineoplastic	Cancer

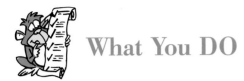

What You DO

When infusing a vesicant, the insertion site and the vein must be closely monitored. If an extravasation is suspected, act immediately. Stop the infusion and clamp off the line. Disconnect the tubing from the catheter, attach an empty 3-cc syringe directly to the catheter, and withdraw as much of the medication (e.g., chemotherapy) into the syringe from the catheter. Then, discontinue the IV catheter. Current research states that care will include steroids, ice, and raising the extremity. For docetaxel, dilute the chemotherapy that is extravasated with subcutaneous saline $\times$ 1, apply ice packs for 30 minutes, and apply topical dimethylsulfoxide (DMSO) $\times$ 3 every 45 minutes.

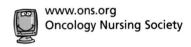

www.ons.org
Oncology Nursing Society

Vesicant Drugs—cont'd

MEDICATION	CLASSIFICATION	USES
Mechlorethamine	Antineoplastic	Cancer
Mitomycin	Antineoplastic	Cancer
Nitroprusside sodium	Antihypertensive, vasodilator	Hypertensive crisis, acute congestive heart failure, cardiogenic shock
Norepinephrine	Adrenergic, catecholamine	Acute hypotension, shock
Paclitaxel	Antineoplastic	Cancer
Platinol	Antineoplastic	Cancer
Promethazine (Phenergan)	Antihistamine, H1-receptor antagonist, phenothiazine derivative	Allergy symptoms, nausea, rhinitis, sedation
Sodium bicarbonate	Alkalinizer	Metabolic acidosis, cardiac arrest, urinary alkalinization, antacid
Vinblastine	Antineoplastic	Cancer
Vincristine	Antineoplastic	Cancer
Vinorelbine	Antineoplastic	Cancer
10%, 20%, or 50% dextrose	Caloric	Increase caloric intake, increase fluid intake

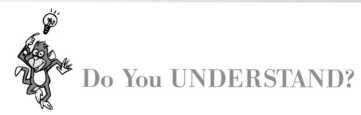

Do You UNDERSTAND?

DIRECTIONS: **Fill in the blanks with the appropriate response.**

1. Another name for tissue death in tissue is _____.

2. When tissue falls off of the body it is said to be _____ off.

DIRECTIONS: **Name a medication that is a potential vesicant in each of the following categories.**

3. Used in radiology departments: _____

4. Antiemetic: _____

5. Dextrose solution: _____

6. Cardiac stimulant, vasopressor: _____

7. Antihypertensive: _____

DIRECTIONS: **Place the number "1" next to the FIRST nursing interventions to be done during an extravasation and the number "2" next to the second nursing interventions to be done, and then a 3, 4, and 5, respectively.**

8. _____ Withdraw medication into syringe.
9. _____ Attach syringe to the IV catheter hub.
10. _____ Clamp off IV line.
11. _____ Discontinue IV catheter.
12. _____ Disconnect the IV tubing from the IV catheter.

What IS Phlebitis?

Phlebitis is an inflammation of the vein wall. Recognized as the most common IV complication, phlebitis can occur during the course of IV therapy or 48 to 96 hours after a catheter is removed (postinfusion phlebitis).

What You NEED TO KNOW

Signs and symptoms of phlebitis include pain, redness (erythema), edema, or any combination. A palpable cord (feels similar to a piece of cord) is felt with severe phlebitis. Pain is often the first sign of phlebitis. When the lining of a vein is damaged, an inflammatory response begins, causing the redness, tenderness, and possibly warmth at the site of the damage. Additionally, capillary permeability increases and fluids move into the interstitial space, causing edema and tenderness. Immunocompromised patients may not be able to respond to vein damage with the traditional symptoms, even though vein wall damage is present.

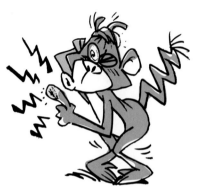

The causative agent that damages the vein categorizes phlebitis. There are three causative agents: mechanical, chemical, and bacterial.

- **Mechanical phlebitis** results when the catheter is the causative agent. The red streak is seen at the insertion site and over the catheter track (see color plate 8).

- **Chemical phlebitis** results when the infusate is the causative agent. The osmolarity or the pH is significantly different from that of blood. With hyperosmolar drugs, the cells lining the vein wall shrink and crack as fluid is pulled into the blood to dilute the infusate. With hypotonic solutions, the cells swell and break as fluid shifts out of the blood into them. Irritant, acidic, or alkalotic drugs burn the cells. The red streak is seen over the vein track (see color plates 9 and 10).

- **Bacterial phlebitis** results when a bacterium is the causative agent. If the patient has a sudden spike in temperature and purulent drainage occurs at the site, bacteria should be suspected as the source. Bacteria are introduced into the IV system either from the IV solution, the tubing, or the catheter. Bacterial phlebitis is rare and is associated with an 18-fold increased risk of IV related septicemia.

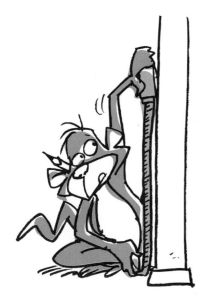

What You DO

Prevention: The best prevention for phlebitis is implementing strategies that will minimize vein wall damage. Think about the patient's potential for phlebitis before IV insertion. If at-risk patients are not identifiable, then measures can be taken to minimize phlebitis occurrence, such as checking with the pharmacy to see if the medication can be diluted in twice as much fluid (if patient is not fluid restricted) or planning to apply warm moist heat to the vein during infusion. Heat promotes venous dilation and increases blood flow, resulting in improved hemodilution. When selecting a catheter, think about optimizing the catheter/vein ratio by choosing the smallest catheter possible and placing it in the largest vein available. If the patient has only small veins and a larger catheter is required for therapy than can be safely inserted, a midline or central line may be best. Avoid bifurcations, hard veins, boney prominences, areas of flexion, and bruises. Do not place tape around the arm. Use securement devices to minimize catheter movement, especially with agitated, confused patients and pediatric patients. Problem-free catheters should be rotated every 96 hours. Rotate large catheters used for surgery or trauma to smaller catheters as soon as possible. To prevent bacterial phlebitis, follow strict aseptic technique, at all times, with every aspect of IV care.

Assessment: It is important to assess the insertion site and the entire venous track. Palpate the site for signs of tenderness. Ask the patient about the presence of pain. Pain is often the first sign of phlebitis.

Treatment: The IV must be discontinued at the first sign of phlebitis. If the IV is not discontinued, the phlebitis will only worsen. When bacterial phlebitis is suspected, the insertion site and the catheter tip should be cultured. If possible, determine the causative agent. When restarting the IV, implement new preventative strategies that were not previously undertaken to prevent new episodes of phlebitis. The best location for the new IV site is in the opposite arm. If this location is not possible, move up the arm at least 3 inches and to the opposite side of the arm. When bacterial phlebitis is suspected, a completely new IV administration setup, including solution, is required. The INS has developed a phlebitis scale to use in assessing and documenting findings.

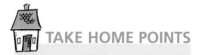

TAKE HOME POINTS

Do not delay routine peripheral catheter rotations with immunocompromised patients.

Phlebitis Scale*

SEVERITY	FINDINGS
0+	No clinical symptoms
1+	Erythema at access site with or without pain
2+	Pain
	Erythema or edema
3+	Pain
	Erythema or edema
	Streak formation
4+	Palpable cord +/−1 inch
	Pain at access site with erythema
	Streak formation
	Palpable venous cord >1 inch
	Purulent drainage

*If this scale is not being used in an institution, then the description associated with the number can be used to describe the assessment.

TAKE HOME POINTS

- The vein damage causative agent determines the phlebitis type.
- Selecting the largest vein and choosing the smallest catheter that will deliver the prescribed flow rate minimizes phlebitis potential.

What IS Thrombophlebitis?

Thrombophlebitis is the presence of inflammation of a vein (phlebitis) and a blood clot (thrombus) on the vein wall.

What You NEED TO KNOW

Clot (thrombus) formation is an extension of phlebitis. Thrombosis is a more common complication with central venous catheters (CVCs). (See Chapter 5 for more information.) As a clot becomes larger in a peripheral vein, it will feel hard. Sometimes, when the catheter is removed, the clot formation will continue, and the vein will completely close (stenosis). A hard lump may be felt or seen (or both). The signs of phlebitis will also be present.

TAKE HOME POINTS

- Venous thrombosis is often invisible until the infusion rate slows or leaking at the site occurs.
- Superficial thrombophlebitis is not to be confused with deep vein thrombosis, which involves deep veins.

Risk Factors

- Poor catheter/vein ratio
- Catheters placed in small vein tributaries instead of main channels (Blood flows through path of least resistance [larger vein] and bypasses the small vein causing stasis.)
- Catheter tips placed just below vein bifurcations
- Catheters placed over boney prominences or areas of flexion
- Extremely low gravity infusion rates (e.g., <20 ml/hr)

What You DO

Prevention: The best methods for preventing thrombus formation are to minimize vein wall damage (same as with phlebitis) and venous stasis (proper catheter/vein ratio). Patients with poor venous access should have a CVC placed instead of repeated peripheral catheter placement. Pumps should be used with low infusion rates. Know the type of needleless cap system that is being used. Always maintain positive pressure on the syringe barrel and close clamp before disconnecting with nonpositive pressure caps. This minimizes reflux of blood back into the catheter. Remember, this procedure is not necessary with positive pressure caps.

Treatment: The IV must be discontinued when thrombosis is suspected. Notify the physician if infection is suspected.

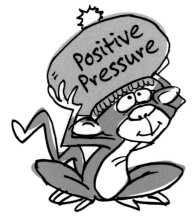

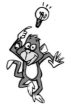

Do You UNDERSTAND?

DIRECTIONS: **Identify the following statements as** *true* **(T) or** *false* **(F).**

1. _____ Inflammation of the vein wall in called infiltration.
2. _____ Phlebitis is the most common IV complication.
3. _____ Phlebitis can occur up to 96 hours after an IV catheter is removed.
4. _____ Petechiae is a common symptom of phlebitis.

Answers: 1. F, phlebitis; 2. T; 3. T; 4. F.

DIRECTIONS: **Match the type of phlebitis in Column A with the cause in Column B.**

Column A

5. _____ Mechanical phlebitis
6. _____ Chemical phlebitis
7. _____ Bacterial phlebitis

Column B

a. Associated with IV septicemia
b. Infusate is causative agent
c. Catheter is causative agent

DIRECTIONS: **Fill in the blanks for each statement as it relates to the prevention of phlebitis.**

8. Always use the smallest catheter in the _____ vein.

9. Problem-free catheters should be rotated every _____ hours.

10. Place new catheters at least _____ inches above the old insertion site.

11. Avoid bifurcations, hard veins, and _____ prominences when placing catheters.

DIRECTIONS: **Match the causes in Column A with the effects in Column B regarding thrombophlebitis.**

Column A

12. _____ Clot grows
13. _____ Retrograde flow of infusate
14. _____ Catheter removed and vein

Column B

a. Stenosis
b. Increases venous stasis
c. Leaking at insertion site closes

DIRECTIONS: **Fill in the blanks with the appropriate response.**

15. The primary treatment for thrombophlebitis is discontinuation of the

   _____.

16. Apply _____ compresses to a phlebitic site.

17. If there is phlebitis in the right arm of an adult, then the nurse should first try to restart the IV in the _____

   _____.

What IS a Hematoma?

A hematoma is uncontrolled bleeding at the insertion site that forms a painful lump. A hematoma occurs most often at the time of insertion or with catheter removal (see color plates 11 and 12).

What You NEED TO KNOW

The initial lump that is formed by the uncontrolled bleeding will dissipate. The rate of decrease depends on the amount of subcutaneous tissue present between the vein and the skin surface. As the blood moves out into the tissue, a bruised (ecchymotic) area forms. Pain is greatest when the induration is the greatest. Patients at risk of hematoma formation include those with:

- Increased tissue and vein fragility
- Anticoagulant therapy
- Long-term steroid therapy
- Renal failure
- Diabetes mellitus
- Advanced age

Hematomas are usually caused by:

- Poor venipuncture technique; the catheter punctures the back wall of the vein.
- Too tight tourniquet application; the vein bursts when needle is inserted.
- Insufficient pressure application during catheter removal; this is especially true with anticoagulated patients.

TAKE HOME POINTS

Anticoagulants that may cause hematoma include heparin, Coumadin, NSAIDs, Plavix, and aspirin.

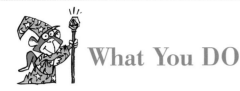

What You DO

Prevention: Identify patients who are at risk for hematoma formation before beginning the venipuncture procedure. No matter what method is used for venous distention, apply with minimal pressure necessary to achieve venous distention. With some older adult patients, using a hand to compress the arm above the potential site may be sufficient.

Treatment: If a hematoma develops during insertion, immediately release the tourniquet and remove the catheter. When a hematoma has occurred, apply light pressure for at least 1 to 2 minutes to the insertion site with a piece of gauze. Check the site to see if bleeding has stopped. Continue holding pressure until bleeding ceases. When bleeding has stopped, apply tape to the gauze. Place a cold compress over the ecchymotic area. Do not use an alcohol pad. Alcohol will slow clotting.

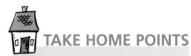

TAKE HOME POINTS

Do not apply a tourniquet above a recent blood draw site because the site can ooze and create a hematoma.

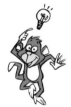

Do You UNDERSTAND?

DIRECTIONS: **Place a plus (+) sign next to the causes of or increased risk factors for hematoma formation.**

1. _____ Catheter punctures back of vein wall.
2. _____ Patient is taking antihypertensive medications.
3. _____ Tourniquet is too tight during venipuncture.
4. _____ Patient is on anticoagulant therapy.
5. _____ Patient has scabies.

DIRECTIONS: **Place a "1" next to the first nursing intervention that should be implemented after a hematoma forms from venipuncture. Then place a "2" next to the second nursing intervention that should be done and a "3" next to the third intervention.**

6. _____ Apply light pressure over the insertion site.
7. _____ Remove catheter.
8. _____ Remove tourniquet.

Answers: 1. +; 2. −; 3. +; 4. +; 5. −; 6. 3; 7. 2; 8. 1.

DIRECTIONS: **Choose the correct word to make the statement true.**

9. To prevent hematoma formation during catheter insertion, once a flash-back is seen, the angle of the catheter should be (raised or lowered).

10. Persons receiving (anticoagulants or antihypertensives) need sufficient pressure applied during catheter removal to prevent the formation of hematoma.

11. Place a (cold or warm) compress over the ecchymotic area of a hematoma as an appropriate nursing intervention.

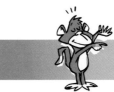

What IS a Site Infection?

A site infection is a localized infection that occurs at the insertion site (see color plate 13).

TAKE HOME POINTS

The insertion site of immunocompromised patients may not be red and indurated because of a decrease in neutrophils.

⚠ **This lack of a response or decreased response to infection is normal for these patients. A minimal response may signal a serious problem.**

What You NEED TO KNOW

A site infection may be identified before or after the IV catheter has been removed. Symptoms are restricted to the skin around the insertion site. The skin will be red, and the insertion site will be swollen (indurated). Drainage may or may not be present. The site will appear similar to the area around a hangnail.

What You DO

⚠ **To prevent infection, maintaining strict aseptic techniques is extremely important in all aspects of IV care.**

Prevention: Maintain strict aseptic technique with all aspects of IV care. Maintain an intact dressing over the insertion site. Dressings should be changed when not intact. If the dressing has been compromised in such a way as to allow air to reach the insertion site, additional tape used to reinforce a loose dressing should be avoided. Instead, change the dressing. The catheter should be stabilized. Catheter movement allows trauma to the insertion site. Trauma causes swelling and increased fluid production around the catheter, increasing the ability of skin bacteria to migrate into the insertion site.

Treatment: The IV catheter must be removed if a site infection is suspected. Drainage (if present) must be cultured. After catheter removal, the site should be cleansed with alcohol and a sterile gauze dressing applied. Notify the physician. A course of the appropriate broad-spectrum antibiotic is commonly prescribed, especially when drainage is severe.

The site should be monitored daily until the infection has resolved. All interventions, site assessments, and patient responses should be documented in the patient's record.

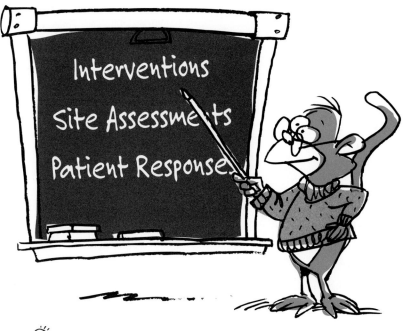

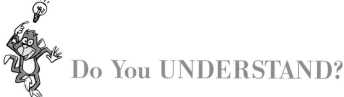 Do You UNDERSTAND?

DIRECTIONS: **Match the causes in Column A with the effects in Column B.**

Column A	Column B
1. _____ Indurated area	a. IV site infection
2. _____ A localized infection	b. Swollen area
3. _____ Catheter movement	c. Increases potential for site infection

Answers: 1. b; 2. a; 3. c.

DIRECTIONS: **Place a plus (+) sign next to the interventions that will decrease IV site infections.**

4. _____ Use aseptic technique during IV care.
5. _____ Change intact dressings every 8 hours.
6. _____ Stabilize IV catheters.
7. _____ Cleanse site area with baking soda every 2 hours.

DIRECTIONS: **Answer the following question.**

8. What overall classification of antibiotic is usually prescribed at the onset of an IV site infection?

_____

CHAPTER 4

Principles of Central Venous Therapy

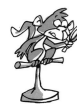

Top Bananas: Chapter 4 Overview

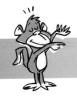

What IS a Central Venous Catheter?

Central venous catheters (CVCs) are catheters with the distal tip that lies in a central vein, usually the superior vena cava (SVC). The increased size of a central vein offers an improved catheter/vein ratio that minimizes vein wall trauma and improves fluid hemodilution.

83

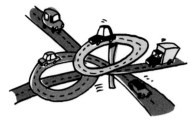

What You NEED TO KNOW

The venous system is similar to a highway system. Smaller peripheral veins lead to larger central veins that lead to the heart. Depending on the insertion site, catheters are threaded through veins until the catheter tip is in the lower one third of the SVC.

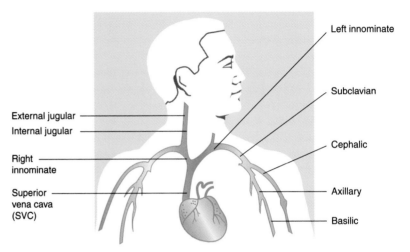

Basilic vein: Located on the inner aspect of the upper forearm and extending into the axillary vein, the basilic vein is the insertion site for arm ports and peripherally inserted central catheters (PICC).

Cephalic vein: Located on the outer border of biceps, then between biceps, pectoralis, and deltoid muscle and curving down to axillary vein, the cephalic vein is smaller compared with the basilic vein. This vein can be used with PICCs that are inserted in the antecubital fossa.

Axillary vein: A peripheral vein that is an extension of basilic vein and terminating beneath clavicle over first rib, the axillary vein extends into the subclavian vein. Catheters inserted into the basilic or cephalic veins travel through this vein.

Subclavian vein: An extension of the axillary vein, the subclavian vein is medial of thoracic inlet and part of the thoracic cavity. This vein is the most common insertion site for CVCs and is the preferred vein for nontunneled CVCs according to the Centers for Disease Control and Prevention (CDC).

Right innominate: An extension of the right subclavian, the right innominate is almost vertical and joins the left innominate just below the first rib and right of the sternum.

Left innominate: An extension of the left subclavian vein, the left innominate has a downward slant that is larger and longer compared with the right innominate.

External jugular veins: Located on the sides of the neck, cannulation of the SVC is not always as successful as it is when accessing the internal jugular.

Internal jugular veins: Both right and left deep veins of the neck and larger than the external jugular, the internal jugular veins have a straight pathway to the SVC. This area is the preferred site for hemodialysis and pheresis according to the CDC.

SVC: This vein carries all the blood from upper one half of the body to the heart and is the extension of the joined innominate veins below the first rib and right of the sternum.

What You DO

If the CVC has not been placed, the chosen insertion site will affect this process. It is important to identify the vein that was used as the insertion site for any CVC. This site affects the development of nursing care and maintenance plan of care. An understanding of the central anatomy will assist the nurse when providing patient education.

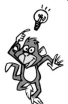

Do You UNDERSTAND?

DIRECTIONS: **Identify the following statements as** *true* **(T) or** *false* **(F).**

1. _____ Smaller peripheral veins lead to larger central veins that lead to the heart.
2. _____ The tip of a correctly placed CVC is in the SVC.
3. _____ The increased size of a central vein offers improved catheter/vein ratio that minimizes vein wall trauma and improves fluid hemodilution.

DIRECTIONS: **Match the vein type in Column A to the definition in Column B.**

Column A

4. _____ External jugular
5. _____ Subclavian vein
6. _____ SVC
7. _____ Cephalic vein

Column B

a. Located on the outer border of the biceps and curves down into the axillary vein; used for PICCs
b. Carries all the blood from the upper one half of the body to the heart
c. Most common insertion site for a CVC
d. Superficial veins on the side of the neck

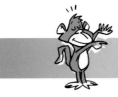

What ARE the Types of Central Venous Catheters?

CVCs are subdivided into three categories based on length of use:

- *Short-term central venous catheters* (STCVCs) are indicated when the duration of therapy is less than 30 days.
- *Intermediate central venous catheters* are indicated for therapy duration of up to 42 days.
- *Long-term central venous catheters* (LTCVCs) or tunneled catheters are indicated when therapy duration is longer than 42 days.

**Groshong®
Distal End Valve**

What You NEED TO KNOW

CVCs are made of either silicone or polyurethane. Silicone is a soft material; it gains its wall strength from wall thickness. Polyurethane is a stiffer material. To make polyurethane soft, the material is made thinner. The internal lumen of silicone catheters is smaller than that of polyurethane catheters of similar gauge (see Chapter 2). The smaller lumen size of silicone catheters results in slower flow rates than those of similar gauge polyurethane catheters. Polyurethane catheters are stronger than silicone catheters and are less prone to damage.

Closed
Neutral pressure

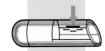

Aspiration
Negative pressure

Infusion
Positive pressure

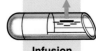

CVCs are also configured with an open tip, a valved distal end (Groshong®, Bard, Salt Lake City, Utah), or valved proximal end (PasV™, Boston Scientific, Natick, Mass). The valved catheters allow fluid to flow in and samples of blood to be removed for laboratory analysis. When the catheter is not in use, the valve is closed, preventing blood reflux that occurs when a patient takes a breath (inspiration). Open-tip catheters must be clamped at all times to prevent the possibility of hemorrhage or air embolism. Valved catheters do not need to be clamped. Heparinized saline flush, as a final instillation, is not necessary in valved catheters. Catheters come in single-, double-, triple- (most common), or quad-lumen configuration.

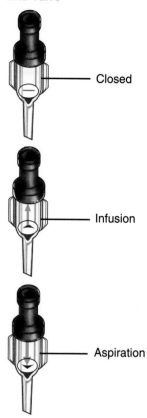

PasV™ Proximal End Valve

— Closed

— Infusion

— Aspiration

What You DO

Determine if the patient has a short-term or long-term catheter. Compare this type of catheter with the current length of therapy and the proposed duration of treatment. For example, a patient with a short-term catheter has been diagnosed with breast cancer and will need a 6-month chemotherapy regimen. For this treatment, a long-term catheter placement might need to be considered during the current hospital stay. Determine whether the catheter material is silicone or polyurethane. This information will affect all areas of nursing care and maintenance plan of care.

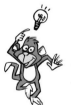

Do You UNDERSTAND?

DIRECTIONS: **Fill in the blanks to complete the statement.**

1. _____-term CVCs are used when therapy is less than 30 days.

2. _____ catheters are stronger than are silicone catheters.

3. _____-tipped catheters must be clamped.

4. Heparin flush is not necessary with _____ catheters.

Answers: 1. Short; 2. Polyurethane; 3. Open; 4. valved.

DIRECTIONS: **Identify the following statements as** *true* **(T) or** *false* **(F).**

5. _____ Short-term catheters can stay in place for up to 1 year.

6. _____ Gauge size alone is a factor in determining flow rate.

7. _____ Valved catheters do not need to be clamped.

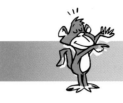

What IS a Short-Term Central Venous Catheter?

STCVCs are commonly used in the inpatient setting. Examples include multilumen subclavian and jugular, dialysis, and pulmonary artery (Swan) catheters.

What You NEED TO KNOW

STCVCs are softer than peripheral intravenous (IV) catheters but are still stiffer compared with a vein or long-term catheters. The potential for vein wall trauma limits dwell time to less than 30 days. The direct access into the vein increases the risk of infection. Ninety percent of all bloodstream infections occur with multilumen subclavian and jugular catheters. There is an estimated 12% to 25% attributable mortality for each infection and a marginal cost of $25,000 per episode. STCVCs can be antimicrobial or antiseptic impregnated. Antimicrobial-antiseptic cuffs can also be applied to the catheter at the time of insertion.

Multilumen catheter: Configurations are designed with extensions (pigtails) for each lumen. The pigtails have staggered lengths. Each pigtail on an open-ended catheter has a slide clamp. Pigtails are covered by a stabilization hub and a single catheter shaft. Each pigtail hub is also color coded to signify lumen outlet location. The gauge size of the lumen is labeled on the hub of each pigtail. Each lumen exit is staggered down the side of the catheter shaft, with one lumen exiting the tip of the catheter shaft. With triple-lumen catheters (the most common configuration), the proximal lumen is located highest on the catheter (longest pigtail), followed by the medial or middle lumen (middle length pigtail), and finally the distal or lowest lumen (short-

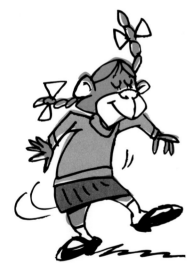

⚠ Color coding is not standardized on CVCs; the nurse must read the manufacturer's information material to be able to identify the exit site location for each lumen.

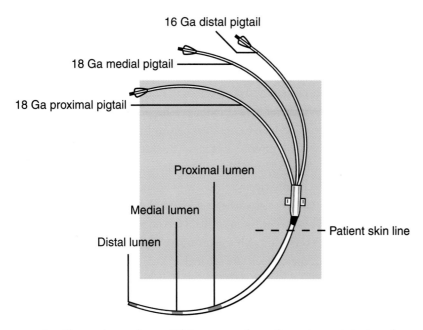

est pigtail) on the catheter. This staggered configuration minimizes drug interaction and allows different procedures (e.g., central venous pressure (CVP) monitoring, blood draw) and different therapies (e.g., electrolyte replacement, antibiotic administration) to be done concurrently. The outside of the catheter shaft is marked in length increments.

Advantages:
- Bedside insertion
- Economical
- Comfortable
- Improved dressing adhesion
- Easily removed
- Easily exchanged over a guide wire

Disadvantages:
- Not designed for long-term use
- Stiff nature of material can cause vein trauma
- Routine care and maintenance
- Potential for spontaneous pneumothorax, hemothorax, or other complications with insertion
- Increased risk of infection, especially with jugular insertion
- Difficult to insert into subclavian vein with obese patients
- Subclavian location contraindicated in patients with chronic obstructive pulmonary disease (COPD)
- Postinsertion x-ray required

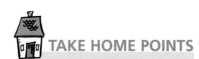

TAKE HOME POINTS

- With triple-lumen catheters, the distal lumen is usually used for CVP monitoring or high-volume infusions, whereas the proximal lumen is typically used for blood draws.
- The more lumens used, the greater the risk for sepsis.

Do not use dialysis catheters for blood draws or other therapies.

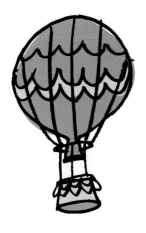

Dialysis catheters: These catheters are used for short-term hemodialysis only and are very large (13 to 16 gauge), which makes them difficult to stabilize and on which to maintain an occlusive dressing.

Pulmonary artery catheter: The Swan catheter is inserted into a central vein (subclavian or jugular) and is advanced until the tip is placed in the pulmonary artery. The catheter is 110 cm long, is heparin coated, and commonly has four lumens. The lumens are attached to hemodynamic monitoring equipment that measures arterial pressure. The distal end of the catheter is surrounded by a balloon. This design allows the catheter to "float" through the right atrium and ventricle and into the pulmonary artery. Once inflated, the balloon maintains correct catheter position and measures pressure from the left side of the heart. The Swan catheter has an additional connector that allows infusions to occur through the introducer sheath. The Swan catheter is used primarily in the critical care setting.

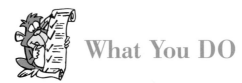

What You DO

It is important for the nurse to understand the risks and benefits of placing a device at a recommended site.

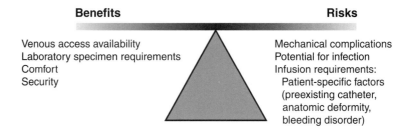

Benefits	Risks
Venous access availability	Mechanical complications
Laboratory specimen requirements	Potential for infection
Comfort	Infusion requirements:
Security	Patient-specific factors
	(preexisting catheter,
	anatomic deformity,
	bleeding disorder)

The most appropriate patient selected for an STCVC:
- Has limited venous access,
- Requires IV therapy less than 30 days
- Requires multiple therapies (e.g., fluids, blood products, multiple medications) and blood draws
- Needs high fluid volume
- Needs any combination of the above

Some therapies, such as vesicants and total parenteral nutrition (TPN) require a central line. Drugs such as irritants, amphotericin B, all penicillins, erythromycin, methicillin, morphine, nafcillin, oxacillin, pentamidine, rocephin, some chemotherapy drugs, and those with extreme pH (e.g., vancomycin) are best given through a central line to minimize peripheral vein damage, especially when being administered over an extended period. Use an STCVC with the minimum number of lumens essential for the prescribed therapy. The use of an antimicrobial- or antiseptic-impregnated catheter in adults is recommended if the patient is at high risk for an infection (e.g., receiving TPN, neutropenic, in intensive care, catheter placement expected to exceed 4 days) and with dialysis catheters with expected usage of more than 2 weeks (according to the CDC). TPN requires a dedicated lumen (rationale: drug incompatibilities, increased risk of infection). Follow the institution's protocol for determining lumen-therapy preference. If no protocol exists, then use the proximal lumen for blood draws and the distal port for CVP monitoring and high-volume infusions.

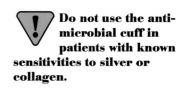

Do not use the anti-microbial cuff in patients with known sensitivities to silver or collagen.

 TAKE HOME POINTS

- Once TPN has been initiated in any lumen, that lumen becomes dedicated to TPN only.
- It is important to keep open-ended catheter pigtail slide clamps, or pinch clamps, in the closed position when a lumen is not in use.

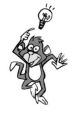

Do You UNDERSTAND?

DIRECTIONS: **Unscramble the words in parentheses to fill in the blanks.**

1. The lumen that is located highest on the subclavian catheter and has the longest pigtail is the _____ lumen. (*rxipolam*)

2. The pigtails of an STCVC are coded by _____. (*lrooc*)

3. TPN and vesicants require the use of a _____ line. (*nctelra*)

DIRECTIONS: **Identify the following statements as *true* (T) or *false* (F).**

4. _____ The potential for spontaneous pneumothorax is a disadvantage of a STCVC.

5. _____ Dialysis catheters should be used for blood draws.

6. _____ Open-ended STCVCs need not be clamped when not in use.

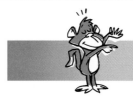

What IS an Intermediate Central Venous Catheter?

The Hohn®, (Bard Vascular Access, Salt Lake City, Utah) is a single-lumen, nontunneled, intermediate CVC.

What You NEED TO KNOW

A Hohn® is made of silicone and has a collagen cuff impregnated with silver ions. The soft silicone material is similar to long-term catheters, allowing the catheter to remain in place for up to 42 days.

Advantages:
- Soft quality of the material minimizes vein wall damage
- Can be used with both inpatient and outpatient populations
- Patient comfort
- Improved dressing integrity
- 5000 U/ml heparin lock every 3 weeks
- Low infection rate
- Bedside insertion

Disadvantages:
- Smaller internal diameter compared with other nontunneled STCVCs; can cause problems with maintaining gravity flow rates of viscous fluid infusions or high infusion rates.

What You DO

Good candidates for a Hohn® catheter are:
- Patients with leukemia who have had difficulty with infections from tunneled lines
- Patients who require central access on a temporary basis
- Terminal patients with no peripheral venous access who require fluids and morphine for comfort measures

- Outpatients on antibiotic or antifungal therapy (i.e., amphotericin therapy)
- Patients with acquired immune deficiency syndrome (AIDS) with less than 6 months' prognosis

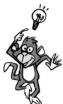

Do You UNDERSTAND?

DIRECTIONS: **Fill in the blanks to complete the statements.**

1. An intermediate catheter can remain in place for _____ to _____ weeks.
2. The _____ material of an intermediate central catheter minimizes trauma to the vein wall.

What IS a Tunneled Catheter?

Tunneled catheters get their name from the method of insertion. The proximal end of the catheter is tunneled under the skin, with the exit site on the chest some distance away from the vein insertion site (entrance site). On the tunneled segment, there is a cuff that forms a barrier under the skin distal to the exit site. The ingrown cuff also stabilizes the catheter and prevents bacteria migration from the exit site into the bloodstream.

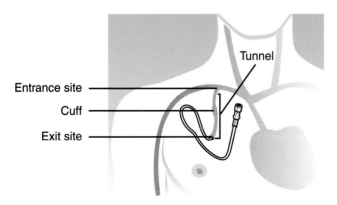

What You NEED TO KNOW

There are two types of tunneled catheters: open-ended and valved. The insertion technique for open-ended and valved catheters is different. Both types of catheters commonly have exit sites on the chest. Open-ended catheters differ primarily in lumen number and size. The Broviac® is single lumen (2.7 to 6.6 Fr) and is used primarily in pediatric patients. The Leonard® is either single or double lumen, and the lumen size is slightly larger than is the smallest Hickman® catheter lumen (10 Fr). The Hickman® catheter is configured single, double, or triple lumen, and the size varies from 9.6 to 14.4 Fr. Valved catheters differ with the placement of the valve. The Groshong® catheter has a distal valve, and the PasV™ has a proximal valve.

Advantages:

- Inserted in outpatient setting
- Easy to repair
- Cuff barrier decreases infection
- Blood sampling
- Multiple lumens
- Requires no special equipment for usage
- Simple removal in outpatient suite or office
- High salvage rate

Disadvantages:

- Postoperative recovery period
- Daily or weekly site and catheter care
- Pinch-off syndrome
- Cost of maintenance supplies
- Altered body image

Contraindications:

- Presence of device-related infection, bacteremia, or septicemia
- Patient's body size insufficient to accommodate the size of the device
- Patient known or suspected to be allergic to materials contained in the device
- Severe chronic obstructive lung disease (percutaneous subclavian placement only)
- Past irradiation of prospective insertion site
- Previous episodes of venous thrombosis or vascular surgical procedures at the prospective placement site
- Local tissue factors preventing proper device stabilization, access, or both

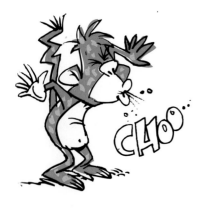

Hickman® and Leonard® Dual Lumen Catheters
(not drawn to scale)

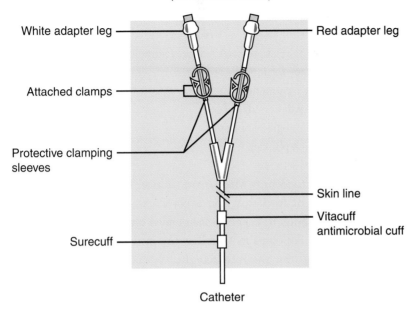

White adapter leg

Attached clamps

Protective clamping sleeves

Surecuff

Red adapter leg

Skin line

Vitacuff antimicrobial cuff

Catheter

Groshong® Catheters
(not drawn to scale)

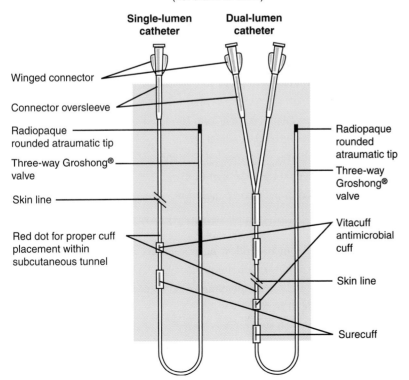

Single-lumen catheter

Dual-lumen catheter

Winged connector

Connector oversleeve

Radiopaque rounded atraumatic tip

Three-way Groshong® valve

Skin line

Red dot for proper cuff placement within subcutaneous tunnel

Radiopaque rounded atraumatic tip

Three-way Groshong® valve

Vitacuff antimicrobial cuff

Skin line

Surecuff

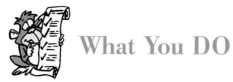

What You DO

The most appropriate patient selected for a tunneled catheter will:
- Require therapy for months or longer
- Require daily treatments
- Be obese, large breasted, or both
- Have a hematologic neoplasm
- Be needle-stick phobic
- Want or need self-care

It is important to identify whether the catheter is open-ended or valved. It is also important to protect the exposed catheter from damage. The catheter should always be capped. Open-ended catheters must be clamped when not in use. For outpatients, follow the institution's policy on maintaining a dressing over the insertion site. With inpatients, an occlusive dressing over the insertion site should be used, which protects the insertion site from nosocomial microorganisms.

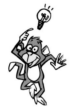

Do You UNDERSTAND?

DIRECTIONS: **Match column A to column B.**

Column A

1. _____	Most common long-term tunneled catheter used in adults
2. _____	Stabilizes the tunneled catheter and prevents bacteria migration
3. _____	Used in pediatric population
4. _____	Requires clamping

Column B

a. Broviac®
b. Hickman®
c. Open-ended catheters
d. Cuff

DIRECTIONS: **All of the following statements are associated with tunneled catheters. Place an "A" for advantage or a "D" for disadvantage next to each statement.**

5. _____ Easy to repair
6. _____ Pinch-off syndrome
7. _____ High salvage rate
8. _____ Blood sampling

Answers: 1. b; 2. d; 3. a; 4. c; 5. A; 6. D; 7. A; 8. A.

What IS an Implanted Port?

Implanted ports are tunneled catheters in which access is under the skin. Unlike other tunneled catheters, there is no external catheter visible. It is important to know that not all implanted ports have the catheter portion located in the SVC. Catheter tips can also be located in the hepatic artery, the peritoneal cavity, and the epidural space. Although the location of venous ports is commonly on the upper chest, they can be located on the lower rib cage. Some venous ports are designed to be implanted underneath the skin of the upper arm. Ports come single and dual lumen, open ended, and distal- or proximal-tip valved.

The physical body location of an implanted port is not indicative of catheter tip location or its reason for usage.

What You NEED TO KNOW

An implanted port has three parts:
1. *Reservoir:* Reservoirs can be made of different material (plastic, stainless steel, titanium) and have different weights, dimensions (high-low profile), and configurations (single-septum, double-septum).
2. *Septum:* A septum covers the reservoir. The entire surface can be punctured for venous access. Septums vary in thickness, diameter, density, and configuration (domed, recessed). Septums are dense enough to hold a needle, are self-sealing, and are designed to be accessed at least 1000 times or more.
3. *Catheter:* The catheter comes either attached to the reservoir (preassembled) from the manufacturer, or they must be attached to the reservoir at the time of insertion. Catheter tips are either open-ended or valved.

PasV™ Port
Proximal Valve

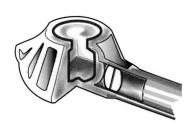

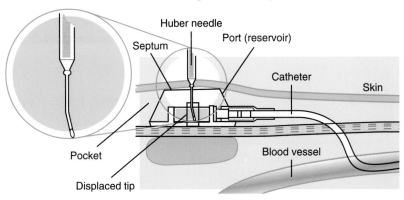

Advantages:
- No interference with activities of daily living
- Better maintenance of body image
- No daily site or catheter care
- Low infection rate (2.5% to 2.7%)

Disadvantages:
- Expense
- Extended postoperative period
- Requires specially designed needle (Huber) for access
- Requires monthly flushing if not in use
- Partial patient disrobing required
- Surgical placement and removal
- Possible needle dislodgment
- Sludge buildup (20% have withdrawal occlusion)
- Possibility of pocket infection
- Pinch-off syndrome
- Significant radiation dose nonconformity with stainless steel type of port
- Must be surgically removed by a physician

Contraindications:
- Presence of device-related infection, bacteremia, or septicemia is known or suspected
- Patient body size insufficient to accommodate the size of the implanted device
- Patient known or suspected to be allergic to materials contained in the device
- Severe chronic obstructive lung disease (percutaneous subclavian catheter placement only; can use peripheral or jugular placement)
- Past radiation therapy to prospective insertion site
- Previous episodes of venous thrombosis or vascular surgical procedures at the prospective placement site
- Local tissue factors preventing proper device stabilization, access, or both

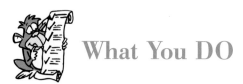 What You DO

The most appropriate patient selected for an implanted port will:
- Require months or longer length of therapy
- Require monthly or cyclic treatments

- Have a solid tumor
- Not want an external reminder
- Be required to have the port to maintain activities of daily living
- Have living conditions that increase the possibility of infection, such as homelessness or poor sanitary living conditions
- Be physically, mentally, or emotionally unable to care for external catheter
- Have limited or inconsistent caregiver availability
- Have equipment and trained nurses available
- Have sufficient means for cost of care

Port Access

Only noncoring needles (Huber) are used to access implanted ports. Traditional needles have a hollow bore that removes some of the septum material (cores); as a result, the septum integrity is permanently damaged and may leak.

Huber needles come in lengths of $^1/_2$ inch, $^3/_4$ inch, 1 inch, and $1^1/_2$ inches. Gauge sizes include 18, 20, and 22. Always choose the smallest gauge needle that will meet the IV therapy requirements and the shortest length that will penetrate the septum completely to enhance patient comfort and dressing adhesion. A winged 90-degree angle Huber needle with attached extension is the common configuration. Needle-protective systems are available.

Preparation: The most important components when accessing a port are asepsis, port stabilization, needle placement in the reservoir, and needle securement.

Palpate the area over the port reservoir to determine the depth, the stability of the reservoir, and the septum location. Palpation will help determine the length of the Huber needle needed to puncture the septum with enough needle length to hit the back of the reservoir. Then the angle of the Huber needle can lay flat on the skin. If the port is deep or is not stable, place something flat and hard (similar to the flat part of a clipboard or thin hard-covered book) behind the chest to give extra support.

Ask the patient about pain that is experienced during access. Patients with older ports may not experience much pain during access. It is best to access a newly placed port during surgery or as soon after surgery as possible if it is to be used during the first week. Normally, the surgical area will swell and be very painful to access for the first week to 10 days. For preexisting ports, assess the skin over and around the septum for inflammation, pain, edema, or exudate. If present, these conditions may signify infection or infiltration. If present, do not access; notify the physician of findings. To minimize pain, a topical or

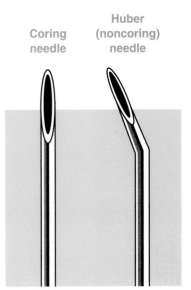

Coring needle   Huber (noncoring) needle

![warning] It is very important to remember that only Huber needles, special noncoring needles, are to be used to access implanted ports. The offset design slices the septum.

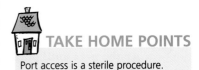

TAKE HOME POINTS

Port access is a sterile procedure.

intradermal lidocaine can be used (see Chapter 2). Another method is to place an ice pack over the site for a few minutes. This technique usually produces enough short-term anesthesia for a painless access procedure.

Procedure:

1. Wash hands and assemble equipment.
2. Carefully unwrap the central line dressing tray. The wrapper of the central line kit becomes the sterile field.
3. Carefully remove the sterile glove packet and mask. Put on the mask.
4. Put one sterile glove on the dominant hand. With the gloved hand, pick up the syringe.
5. With the ungloved hand, pick up the saline bottle. Fill syringe and place on the sterile field.
6. Apply the second glove.
7. Prime the Huber needle and close clamp on the extension.
8. Clean the skin with the skin disinfectants according to institution protocol.
9. Immobilize the port with the index finger and thumb of the nondominant hand.
10. The port septum will be located between these two fingers. Move the fingers to confirm septum location and to determine if there is any septum movement.
11. Extend the fingers to stretch the skin over the septum and to stabilize the reservoir.
12. With the needle perpendicular to the septum, between these two fingers, in one movement, firmly push the needle through the skin and septum until the needle makes contact with the back of the reservoir. This action will require some force. The septum will feel stiff. When the needle is in proper position, the nurse will feel metal against metal, which occurs when the needle hits the back of the reservoir. This contact must be felt to confirm proper placement of the needle.
13. Rotate the wings so that the extension points down the chest or toward the sternum (not toward the arm). This position minimizes needle movement with arm movement.
14. Attach the saline-filled, 10-cc syringe to the cap, open the clamp, and aspirate blood to assess for proper functioning. If there is no blood return, have the patient cough, change position, or both. Attempt to aspirate again. If a blood return is not achieved, flush slightly to assess patency. Attempt to aspirate again.
15. If a blood return is not achieved, proper port functioning and tip location will have to be determined before usage.

TAKE HOME POINTS

It is important to rotate the Huber needle insertion site within the port system to maximize septum life.

TAKE HOME POINTS

Having the patient raise his or her arms over the head, cough, or turn the head to one side or the other sometimes aids in obtaining a positive blood aspirate from a port.

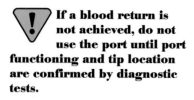

If a blood return is not achieved, do not use the port until port functioning and tip location are confirmed by diagnostic tests.

16. Once a blood return has been established, flush the catheter according to institution protocol.
17. If the port is to remain accessed, a dressing must be applied to stabilize the Huber needle and protect the insertion site from microorganisms. If the Huber needle lies flat against the chest, place a piece of tape across the wings and apply the sterile dressing. Gauze may be used under the wings to provide padding if a space is present.

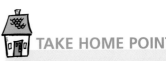

TAKE HOME POINTS

To maintain patency, implanted ports must be flushed with saline, followed by final heparinized saline flush every 4 weeks when not in use.

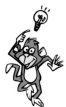

Do You UNDERSTAND?

DIRECTIONS: **Fill in the blanks with the correct answer.**

1. Name the three parts of an implanted port.

   _____

   _____

   _____

2. _____ is a special type of noncoring needle used to access implanted ports.

3. A newly implanted port site is usually sore and painful for up to _____ days.

DIRECTIONS: **Place the number "1" next to the first intervention a nurse would do to access a port, a number "2" next to the second intervention, and so forth, until the last intervention is the number "6."**

4. _____ Prime Huber needle and clamp extension closed.
5. _____ Apply sterile gloves.
6. _____ Cleanse patient skin.
7. _____ Unwrap central line dressing tray.
8. _____ Push needle into septum.
9. _____ Wash hands.

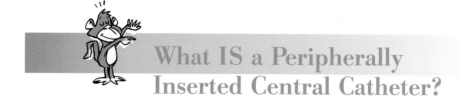

What IS a Peripherally Inserted Central Catheter?

A PICC is inserted into a large peripheral vein in the antecubital space or upper arm, hence the name peripherally inserted.

What You NEED TO KNOW

PICCs are made of silicone or polyurethane. One type is silver-impregnated to minimize the potential for infection. PICCs come in single-, double-, or triple-lumen, open-tipped, or valved configurations (Proximal tip PasV™, and distal end Groshong®). The manufactured length of PICCs can range from 55 to 65 cm. The portion of a PICC that resides in a vein, on average, is 52 cm in length. PICCs are as much as 20 times longer than are peripheral catheters. It is important to understand how the additional length of PICCs and the different catheter materials affect IV therapy activities (see Chapter 2). The product information can identify the original length of the catheter but not the amount that may have been trimmed before insertion.

Advantages:
- Bedside insertion by a specially trained registered nurse or physician
- Economical
- Eliminates risks associated with neck, chest, femoral insertions
- Extremely low infection rate
- Easy to access (makes possible self-administration)
- Easy to remove by a specially trained nurse or physician
- No needle stick required when accessing

Disadvantages:
- Daily care and maintenance (flushing)
- External catheter
- Altered body image
- Potential for mechanical phlebitis
- Requires postinsertion x-ray to verify placement
- Small-gauge silicone PICCs not recommended for blood sampling
- Limits activities of daily living (swimming, bathing); restricts arm mobility
- Requires specially trained nurses or physicians to insert

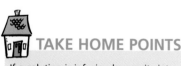

TAKE HOME POINTS

If a solution is infusing by gravity into an adult patient through a PICC line, the flow will be slower than the same fluid flowing through a 1-inch peripheral catheter of similar gauge.

- Require pump to achieve a flow rate on some small-gauge silicone PICCs
- Possible damage to external portion of the catheter

Contraindications:

- Preexisting skin infection
- Uncooperative, confused patient (can pull out)
- Anatomic distortions of venous pathway
- Severe peripheral edema

TAKE HOME POINTS

- Small-gauge silicone PICCs do not have sufficient flow rates for patients who require high-volume infusions. It is important to know the flow capabilities of a patient's PICC.
- PICCs are not recommended for high-pressure infusions, such as those required with computed tomography (CT) scans.

What You DO

The appropriate patient for a PICC will:

- Require therapy greater than 6 days but less than 1 year
- Require daily IV access
- Present chest injuries
- Require radical neck dissection surgery
- Have head or neck cancer
- Present the possibility of independent self-care

PICC is a generic name for 11 different devices currently being marketed today. Although these devices have similarities, they also have differences. It is important to know the type of PICC that a patient had inserted to develop an appropriate plan of care. A PICC has at least 1 inch of visible external catheter between the insertion site and the hub. Care must be taken to prevent damage to the catheter.

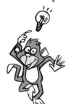
Do You UNDERSTAND?

DIRECTIONS: **Fill in the blanks to complete the statements.**

1. PICC is an abbreviation for _____

_____ _____ catheter.

2. One advantage of a PICC is that it has a low _____

_____.

Answers: 1. peripherally inserted central; 2. infection rate.

3. Some small-gauge silicone PICCs require a _____

_____ to achieve a flow rate.

DIRECTIONS: **Place an "A" for advantage or a "D" for disadvantage next to each statement below. All statements are associated with PICCs.**

4. _____ Altered body image
5. _____ No needle sticks required for accessing
6. _____ Bedside insertion
7. _____ Daily flushing

What IS Insertion?

Insertion is the procedure that results in the catheter being placed into the human body. Physicians insert nontunneled, tunneled, implanted, and PICCs. Specially trained nurses insert PICCs. Informed consent must be obtained before catheter insertion. After insertion, all catheters tip locations must be verified by x-ray before use.

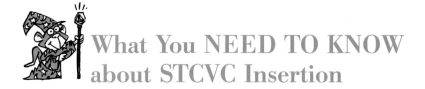

What You NEED TO KNOW about STCVC Insertion

Insertion is a sterile procedure performed by a physician. The CDC recommends that full barrier precautions be followed during insertion (gloves, mask for both the inserter and assistant personnel, gown, head cover, large body covering drape for the patient's chest and lower body, and screening the tracheostomy or **T** tube with a drape to act as a barrier between it and the insertion site). Local anesthesia is used. The Seldinger method is used with insertion, which includes a percutaneous insertion with a large needle into the chosen vein, a guide wire being advanced through the needle, the needle being removed, a dilator being passed over the guide wire and advanced to enlarge the vein opening, the dilator being removed, the catheter being passed over the guide wire into the SVC to appropriate marking on the catheter, the guide wire being removed, and each pigtail being aspirated for a blood return and then flushed with saline. The catheter is sutured on the suture wings to prevent inadvertent removal and to maintain correct tip placement. A postinsertion placement x-ray is required to determine tip location before any infusion is initiated.

What You DO

The nurse's responsibilities include collecting equipment, preparing a clean work site (cleaning the bed table, removing all clutter), having patient void before the procedure, getting the patient comfortable, removing any clothing over insertion site, and cleaning the skin (at least 6-inch square) with soap and water. If the patient has a hairy chest, shave (with an electric shaver) the potential insertion area (6-inch square on the chest) or clip hair on the neck and shave face where the dressing will be placed. If the femoral site is to be used, shave the area.

Assess vital signs. The physician may want the patient to be placed in Trendelenburg position just before insertion to decrease the potential for air embolism. Know how to place the bed in Trendelenburg position. During the time of actual needle puncture, the physician may want the patient to perform a Valsalva maneuver. Teach the patient (before the procedure) to take a deep breath, hold it, and bear down. Have the patient return the demonstration of the Valsalva maneuver if medically appropriate.

During the procedure, the physician may want the nurse to aspirate blood to assess for tip placement and flush each lumen. Once the line has been sutured, it usually is the nurse's responsibility to dress the site with a sterile dressing and appropriately dispose of all the insertion equipment and all sharps in a sharps container.

Notify the physician immediately if:

- Bleeding occurs at the insertion site, creating more than a 2" × 2" bloody area. Be sure to reinforce the dressing.
- Signs of pneumothorax (shortness of breath, absent or diminished breath sounds on the affected side) develop.
- Cyanosis is present.
- Hematoma or bruising develops on the chest wall.

When shaving, straight-edge razors should be avoided. This type of razor can cause nicks that can become infected.

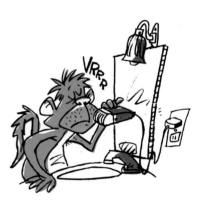

A return demonstration of the Valsalva maneuver should not be done in patients with a cardiac history (rationale: cardiac stimulation and bradycardia may result).

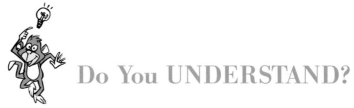

Do You UNDERSTAND?

DIRECTIONS: **Choose the one correct answer in parentheses for each statement.**

1. An STCVC is inserted using _____ anesthesia. *(local or general)*

2. Postinsertion placement of an STCVC is assessed by _____. *(x-ray or barium contrast)*

3. Remove excess chest, neck, or face hair before STCVC insertion with a(n) _____. *(razor or electric shaver)*

DIRECTIONS: **The CDC recommends full barrier precautions to be followed during insertion.**

4. Which of the following barriers are required? *(Circle all barriers required.)*

   Gloves

   Mask for the inserter

   Mask for assistant personnel

   Gown

   Head cover

   Large body covering drape for the patient's chest and lower body

   Drape to screen the tracheostomy or T tube

DIRECTIONS: **Fill in the blanks to complete the statement.**

5. Teaching the patient to take a deep breath and bear down is teaching the

   _____   _____.

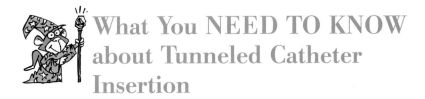

What You NEED TO KNOW about Tunneled Catheter Insertion

Tunneled catheters are placed by physicians in outpatient surgery, radiology, or in the OR under either local or general anesthesia. A cut-down is made near the subclavian vein (entrance site), and an exit site incision is made 2 to 12 inches down the chest wall in the subcutaneous tissue. With open-ended catheters, a special piece of equipment tunnels from the entrance site to the exit site and pulls the catheter up through the tunnel to the entrance site. The catheter is cut to the correct length and threaded into the SVC. A valve-ended catheter is not able to have the distal tip cut. Therefore the procedure is reversed. The catheter is threaded into the SVC. The tunnel is made from the exit site to the entrance site and the catheter is pulled down and out the exit site. The proximal end is then cut to the desired length, and the hubs are added to the lumens. Tip placement is confirmed by x-ray. The catheter may or may not be sutured in place, though suturing is recommended.

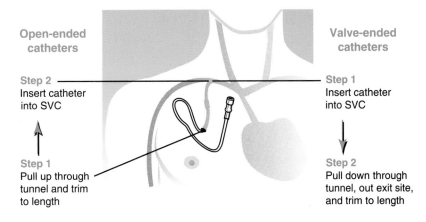

Open-ended catheters

Step 2
Insert catheter into SVC

Step 1
Pull up through tunnel and trim to length

Valve-ended catheters

Step 1
Insert catheter into SVC

Step 2
Pull down through tunnel, out exit site, and trim to length

What You DO

The postinsertion patient will have two catheter placement–related wounds: entrance and exit. The entrance site will usually be closed with Steri-Strips but may also be closed with sutures or metal clips. The tunneled track will be tender and may be bruised.

TAKE HOME POINTS

Cold for the first **24 hours** followed by heat applied to the catheter track will minimize discomfort after tunneled catheter insertion.

Teach the patient to:
- Notify the physician if the site is red, swollen, or has bloody or liquid drainage.
- Keep the site completely dry for the first 24 hours. Resume bathing normally after Steri-Strips have fallen off on their own.

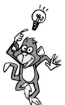

Do You UNDERSTAND?

DIRECTIONS: **Choose the one correct answer in parentheses for the following statement.**

1. A tunneled catheter has both an entrance wound and an
_____ wound site. (*exit* or *air pocket*)

DIRECTIONS: **Fill in the blanks to complete the statements.**

2. Open-ended tunneled catheters are pulled _____
through the exit site, cut, and then threaded through the entrance
site into the SVC.

3. Valve-tunneled catheters are pulled from the entrance site
_____ out the exit site and then
cut to the correct length.

4. The application of _____ for the
first 24 hours followed by _____ applied
to the catheter track will minimize discomfort after tunneled catheter
insertion.

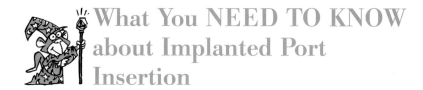

What You NEED TO KNOW about Implanted Port Insertion

Implanted ports are placed by surgeons in outpatient surgery or the OR or by interventional radiologists using local anesthesia. The subclavian or jugular vein is cannulated by cut-down. The port catheter is advanced into the

Answers: 1. exit; 2. up; 3. down; 4. cold, heat.

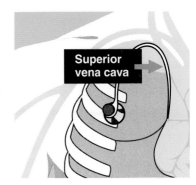

Superior vena cava

SVC. For catheters that are preattached to the port reservoir, the distal tip is trimmed to the correct length before cannulation. For catheters that are not preattached to the port reservoir, the catheter is trimmed at the proximal end after cannulation and attached to the port. A pocket is made on the chest wall above the breast and over a rib or on the dorsal area of the upper arm. The port reservoir is placed in this pocket and sutured into place. The pocket is sutured or steri-stripped closed.

What You DO

Similar to tunneled catheters, there will be two catheter placement–related incisions to monitor (pocket closure and catheter insertion). Complete healing takes 10 days to 2 weeks. The area over the port pocket may swell. Ice pack application for the first 24 hours may minimize edema.

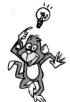

Do You UNDERSTAND?

DIRECTIONS: **Choose the one correct answer in parentheses for the following statement.**

1. To secure an implanted port in the pocket of the chest wall, the reservoir is _____ into place. (*taped or sutured*)

DIRECTIONS: **Identify the following statements as *true* (T) or *false* (F).**

2. _____ Implanted ports can be placed by interventional radiologists.
3. _____ Ultrasound is used to help place implanted ports.
4. _____ Complete healing of the port pocket takes 10 days to 2 weeks.

Answers: 1. sutured; 2. T; 3. F; 4. T.

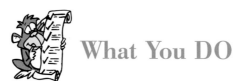

What You NEED TO KNOW about PICC Insertion

At the time of insertion, PICCs may be trimmed to a specific length determined by the approximate venous pathway between the insertion site and the SVC. Direct venipuncture into the vein with an introducer is the common method for vein access. A modified Seldinger method can also be used to access the vein. The modified Seldinger method must be used when bedside ultrasound is being used for placement. Once the vein is accessed, the catheter is passed through the introducer and threaded into the SVC. It is recommended that at least 1 inch of the catheter is not threaded into the vein. This portion forms a dead space between the hub and the insertion site and minimizes trauma to the site with arm movement. The PICC hub must be stabilized to minimize catheter movement that may result in insertion site trauma. Because the introducer makes a larger hole in the vein than does the PICC catheter, when the introducer is removed, the vein does not form a tight fit around the PICC. Twenty four hours is required for the vein to heal around the PICC. During this period, the insertion site might ooze, or some small amount of bleeding can occur. The insertion site and the PICC up to the hub are covered by a pressure dressing.

Do not insert a PICC into the arm of the operative site of a postmastectomy patient or a renal failure patient who is a candidate for an arterio-venous fistula.

What You DO

The initial pressure dressing is changed after 24 hours and replaced with a transparent dressing with no gauze so that the insertion site can be observed. When caring for a patient with a newly inserted PICC, it is important to limit activity of the arm for the first 48 to 72 hours to minimize the potential for mechanical phlebitis. Heat is commonly applied to the upper arm anywhere from 20 minutes (3 to 4 times per day) to continuously for 2 to 3 days after insertion, depending on the institution's protocol. It is important to develop a plan of care for protecting the PICC catheter from damage. This plan might include using a securement device such as StatLock (see color plate 2). Because the insertion site must be protected from water, a plan must be developed to keep the site dry, such as teaching the patient to wrap the site in plastic wrap during bathing.

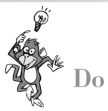

Do You UNDERSTAND?

DIRECTIONS: Choose the one correct answer in parentheses for each statement.

1. Arm activity is limited for up to 72 hours after a _____ is inserted. (*femoral port* or *PICC*)

2. Initial pressure dressing applied at time of insertion is changed at _____. (*24 hrs* or *7 days*)

3. _____ is applied to the upper arm anywhere from 20 minutes, 3 to 4 times per day, to continuously for 2 to 3 days after insertion, depending on the institution's protocol. (*Heat* or *Cold*)

DIRECTIONS: Identify the following statements as *true* (T) or *false* (F).

4. _____ An x-ray is used to verify PICC placement.

5. _____ The initial pressure dressing on a PICC is left on for 72 to 96 hours.

6. _____ It is appropriate to insert a PICC into the arm of the operative site of a postmastectomy patient or a renal failure patient who is a candidate for an arteriovenous fistula.

7. _____ The insertion site, the PICC, and the hub are covered by a pressure dressing throughout PICC use.

What IS Dressing Management?

Management of a CVC dressing requires integrating knowledge about the patient (e.g., immunocompromised, presence of tracheostomy or T tube, excessive coughing, contractures of the neck), the type of organisms that can populate the skin around the insertion site, where the insertion site is located, and how the catheter and the insertion track enhance infection, as well as antiseptics, sterile techniques, and types of dressings.

Answers: 1. PICC; 2. 24 hours; 3. Heat; 4. T; 5. F; 6. F; 7. F.

Purpose of a dressing:
- To minimize insertion site trauma
- To keep the insertion site dry and clean
- To stabilize the catheter

The goal of successful dressing management is to minimize the potential for catheter-related infection.

What You NEED TO KNOW

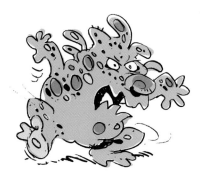

There are three different skin ecosystems: dry (arm), wet (chest, groin), and sebum-rich (jugular). Moisture not only allows bacteria to flourish, but also provides a medium for transit over the skin and down the catheter tract. In addition to *Staphylococcus* epidermis, wet and sebum-rich areas support gram-negative bacilli, fungi, and viruses. The jugular area is close to the nose and mouth and tracheostomy (if present), increasing exposure to a wide variety of bacteria. Because positive-catheter cultures are strongly associated with skin colonization, the goal must be the best possible site preparation to eliminate as many bacteria as possible. (See Chapter 2 for information on skin antiseptics.)

Transparent dressings are commonly used to cover central line insertion sites. These dressings permit observation of the site, act as a barrier to moisture, and are very comfortable. Transparent dressings vary in the amount of moisture that they allow to pass. This characteristic is called the moisture vapor transmission rate (MVTR). The moisture accumulation under different types of transparent dressings can vary a great deal from patient to patient and from brand to brand.

TAKE HOME POINTS

Patients who have fevers or are sweating profusely **(diaphoretic)** may need their transparent dressings changed more frequently compared with the general patient population.

What You DO

The CDC recommends that all dressings should be changed when damp, loosened, or soiled or when inspection of the insertion site is necessary. CVC dressings on adult patients should be routinely changed every 7 days for transparent dressings, every 2 days for gauze dressings, or according to the institution's policy. Pediatric patients are an exception because the risk of dislodging the catheter outweighs the benefit of routine dressing changes.

TAKE HOME POINTS

Always remove the dressing from the catheter hub toward the insertion site to prevent pulling out the catheter. Never use scissors to remove tape or the dressing to prevent accidentally cutting the catheter. Always avoid tension on the catheter.

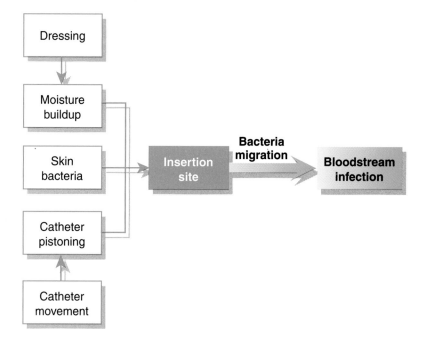

When a transparent dressing is intact around the outside of three edges but is loose over the extension and catheter hub area, do not reinforce the area with tape. Instead, change the dressing according to the institution's standardized procedure for changing central line dressings.

Sterile technique must be maintained throughout the dressing change procedure. Meticulous attention to each step is important. The insertion site and the skin that will be under the dressing should be thoroughly cleaned. Unlike the skin preparation for a peripheral venipuncture, the area to be cleaned is not intact (insertion site and catheter present). The area to be cleaned is larger than that with peripheral catheter preparation. Clean at least a 4- to 6-inch area, with the area being slightly larger than the dressing to be used. Clean starting at the insertion site and work outward. This technique is particularly important to prevent carrying bacteria from the skin back to the insertion site. When using alcohol and iodophor, three swabs of each are used instead of the one of each, as used with peripheral insertions. The insertion site and the exposed catheter hub, as well as the skin, should be cleaned with alcohol. All dry blood should be removed because the presence of organic secretions *negates the antimicrobial action of the iodophor*. If using chlorhexidine preparation or other one-step product, completely wet the same area using friction and working from the insertion site outward. Allow all preparation solutions to dry completely before continuing.

⚠️ **Do not fan, blow on, or blot the area because bacterial kill will be decreased.**

⚠️ **Solutions containing acetone may degrade catheter material and should be avoided.**

Do not use chlorhexidine patches in neonates less than 7 days of age or gestational age less than 26 weeks (according to the CDC).

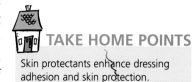

TAKE HOME POINTS
Skin protectants enhance dressing adhesion and skin protection.

Develop an age-appropriate and patient-centered plan for bathing that will minimize the chances of getting the catheter and dressing wet.

If a patient is at high risk for infection, after cleaning the skin, place a chlorhexidine patch over the insertion site. The patch slowly releases chlorhexidine over a 7-day period.

The CDC strongly advises against routine application of antimicrobial ointment to insertion sites. This practice can cause insertion-site maceration and promote fungal growth. Apply a skin protectant (if not using a combination product that includes one) to minimize skin trauma related to routine dressing changes. Skin protectants also improve dressing adhesion. Allow the skin protectant to dry completely before applying the dressing. After the dressing has been applied, apply reinforcing tape around the catheter to secure the dressing-catheter-skin connection. Label the dressing with the date, initials, and other data specified by the institution.

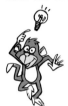

Do You UNDERSTAND?

DIRECTIONS: **Complete the crossword puzzle on the following page.**

Across

1. Technique used to insert a CVC.
3. Isopropyl.
4. Degrades catheters.
6. Abbreviation for the rate at which moisture passes through dressing.
7. Part of catheter that is winged.
9. Risk of dislodging catheter is great in this age group.
10. Type of nontunneled mesh-type dressing used over IVs.

Down

2. Iodine stick.
5. One-step skin preparations for IV.
8. Abbreviation for a peripherally inserted catheter.

Across

1.
3.
4.
6.
7.
9.
10.

Down

2.
5.
8.

DIRECTIONS: **Fill in the blanks to complete the statements.**

11. Cleansing a CVC site should include cleansing at least a _____-inch diameter area.

12. Solutions containing _____ can degrade catheter material and should therefore be avoided around CVCs.

13. If a CVC dressing is wet, the nurse should _____ it.

14. Iodophors require a minimum of _____ minutes of skin contact time to kill bacteria.

What IS Flushing?

Flushing is the displacement of catheter contents (e.g., medications, blood) by pushing a specific amount of fluid (usually saline) through the catheter. The purpose of flushing is to maintain catheter patency. Loss of patency can result in interruption of therapy and possibly even catheter removal. It is important to flush with enough saline to completely displace all the contents of the catheter.

What You NEED TO KNOW

Improper flushing technique can damage the catheter. Silicone catheters are more easily damaged than are polyurethane catheters. The safest way to use syringes with any CVC is to know how the syringe size affects the pressure exerted on the catheter. The relationship between the amount of force used on the syringe plunger and the size of the syringe determines the amount of pressure exerted. When the same force is applied to the plunger of a small syringe, a higher pressure will be generated than when using a larger syringe.

Factors that influence or alter pressure generated by a syringe include the following:

- Force applied to the plunger
- Size of syringe
- Presence or absence of a needle on the end of the syringe
- Resistance generated as a result of the length and gauge size of CVC (greatest with small-gauge PICCs)
- Viscosity of the fluid in the syringe

It is important to understand that the presence of some type of occlusion in the vein or the catheter also increases the resistance felt during the flushing procedure. A partial occlusion, such as a venous spasm or muscle contraction over the catheter track, can occur at any time. For example, if a PICC or arm port is located in the cephalic vein, whenever the surrounding muscles are flexed, a partial occlusion occurs. The most common response to feeling increased resistance in a CVC is to apply more force to the syringe plunger to overcome the resistance. This action should be avoided when flushing CVCs because of the increased potential for catheter damage.

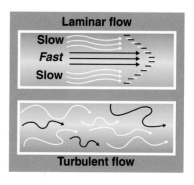

Avoid the temptation of applying more force to the syringe plunger upon feeling increased resistance while flushing CVCs. This will help decrease the potential of catheter damage.

What You DO

The most common size of syringe used for flushing CVCs is a 10-cc syringe. Preservative-free (bacteriostatic) saline is best. If using saline with a preservative, an adult should receive no more than 30 cc of bacteriostatic saline in a 24-hour period because of reactions to the benzyl alcohol preservative in adults. *Flush using a pulsating motion* (rapid repeated push-pause action with the thumb on the plunger of the syringe). This action allows the flush solution to be turbulent, causing the catheter walls to be "scrubbed."

Using a fast steady flushing method initiates laminar flow, which decreases the scrubbing action potential. The fluid in this type of flow is moving rapidly in the center of the stream but slowly at the edge. Think of a river. The water is flowing rapidly down the center but is still along the river edge. Little or no cleaning action is achieved with laminar flow.

Catheters should be flushed with saline before IV administration to determine patency. Flushing should be done slowly and with minimal intermittent pressure. If unusual resistance is felt, *stop*. Do not apply more force to the syringe plunger. Reposition the patient, then have the patient cough and take a deep breath and try to flush again. Never apply force. If resistance continues, first determine the cause before continuing the flushing procedure. After the IV therapy is completed, a final saline flush is implemented to clean the residual solution out of the catheter. This procedure is very important. This final saline flush prevents incompatible solutions from coming into contact with and possibly forming a precipitate in the catheter.

TAKE HOME POINTS

- Always flush with a minimum of 3 to 10 cc before and after each CVC use and 20 cc after blood product administration or blood withdrawal.
- Partial occlusions can occur at any time. Flushing first with a 10-cc syringe to check for patency does not guarantee patency.

If final heparin flush is part of the institution protocol, *follow the saline flush with heparin*. The strength and amount of final heparin flush is determined by the institution protocol. A general rule for a flush volume is:

$$(\text{extension [if added]} + \text{CVC internal volume}) \times 2 = \text{priming volume}$$

For example, if the extension volume is 0.5 cc and the CVC internal volume is 1.0 cc, then the priming volume is:

$$(0.5 \text{ cc} + 1.0 \text{ cc}) \times 2 = 3$$
$$1.5 \text{ cc} \times 2 = 3$$

Normally, 2 to 3 cc of heparinized saline is adequate. The heparin strength varies between 10 and 100 units. Usually, the lower strength is used when the catheter is being used regularly on an intermittent basis (e.g., every 12 hours). The 100 units might be used with patients who are at increased risk for thrombosis or when the catheter is not being used on a regular basis.

When disengaging the syringe from the CVC with nonpositive pressure caps, maintain positive pressure on the syringe plunger, and close clamp on the extension set before disengaging to minimize blood reflux into the catheter. Blood reflux can cause fibrin buildup in the internal lumen of the catheter. Reflux of blood into the distal tip of a catheter on removal of a syringe is a well-known cause of clotted CVCs (see Chapter 5). Maintaining pressure on the plunger creates positive pressure within a catheter at the conclusion of flushing, rather than allow a vacuum to develop, pulling blood into the end of the catheter. Do not close the clamp before syringe removal with positive pressure caps.

If the flushing procedure is done improperly or with an insufficient amount of flush solution, loss of patency can occur.

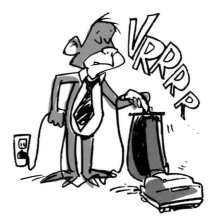

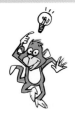

Do You UNDERSTAND?

DIRECTIONS: **Match Column A with Column B.**

Column A

Column B

1. _____ Common syringe for flushing CVCs

a. 2 to 3 cc

2. _____ Maximum amount of bacteriostatic saline
for flushing, in an adult, within a 24-hour
period with a CVC

b. 20 cc

c. 30 cc

d. 10 cc

3. _____ Amount of heparinized saline used in CVCs
to prevent occlusion or to ease flow

4. _____ Minimum amount of saline flush to use with
blood products

DIRECTIONS: **Identify the following statements as *true* (T) or *false* (F).**

5. _____ Muscle flexing can cause a partial occlusion of a PICC that is
in the cephalic vein.

6. _____ Force applied to a syringe plunger does not alter pressure.

7. _____ If resistance is felt when flushing a PICC, the next nursing
intervention is to flush harder by pushing harder on the
syringe plunger.

8. _____ Positive pressure should be maintained when disengaging a
syringe from a CVC that has a nonpositive pressure cap.

What IS Blood Withdrawal?

Blood withdrawal is the collecting of blood through a CVC for purposes of
laboratory testing. A CVC is commonly used for collecting laboratory specimens while the CVC is in the patient. Drawing a blood sample requires care
to ensure that the specimens collected will result in reliable findings. It is
important to understand all phases of blood sampling if quality sampling is
to be achieved.

What You NEED TO KNOW

A properly collected blood sample will result in an accurate and reliable test result. A quality specimen is free of hemolysis. Hemolysis occurs when red blood cells are broken as a result of some type of trauma, and the cell contents leak into the plasma. Hemolysis can occur if tubes are vigorously shaken instead of gently rocked, if too little blood is drawn in relation to the additives, or when a blood draw is too rapid, which causes enough turbulence for red blood cell destruction. Hemolysis causes unreliable test results for potassium, sodium, glucose, creatinine, bilirubin, magnesium, and ammonia.

When pulling back on a syringe barrel, less pressure is generated with small syringes than with large ones. This characteristic is opposite from flushing. If the syringe plunger has moved back and an open space with no fluid is present, a vacuum has formed. When this event occurs, blood cannot be withdrawn.

There are two methods used for drawing blood from CVCs: the "vacutainer" method and the syringe-collection method.

Vacutainer method: This system allows the blood being withdrawn to directly fill the specimen tubes. The advantages are as follows:

- Minimal potential exists for exposure to blood.
- Even, consistent pressure exerted during withdrawal decreases the likelihood of hemolysis.
- Tubes automatically fill to exact requirements for preservatives.

The disadvantages are as follows:

- Changing from one tube to another while holding the vacutainer requires technical practice.
- The strength of the vacuum can cause hemolysis, especially with rapid withdrawals.

Syringe-collection method: With this method, the blood is aspirated first into a syringe and then transferred to the specimen tube. The National Committee for Clinical Laboratory Standards (NCCLS) recommends against the use of syringes for blood draws because of the inherent risk of unwanted blood exposure. The advantage is that the amount of pressure and the rate of withdrawal can be more easily controlled.

The disadvantages are as follows:

- This method requires transfer of blood from syringe to the specimen tube, increasing potential for blood exposure.

- A potential exists for overfilling collection tubes.
- A needle for transferring specimen is required.
- The chance of hemolysis when transferring blood from the syringe to the collection tube is increased.

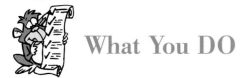

What You DO

Drawing a blood sample requires care to ensure that the specimens collected will result in reliable findings. It is very important to stop all fluids and medications for at least 1 minute before drawing any specimens so as to draw an accurate specimen. Clean the cap with alcohol except if drawing ETOH (ethanol) levels (clean the cap according to institution protocol). Open the clamp and flush the catheter with 10 cc of saline to check for patency and to clean the catheter. Except when drawing blood cultures (no discard required), it is necessary to first draw a sample of blood that will be discarded. This procedure clears the catheter completely, permitting all subsequent draws to be filled only with blood. Withdraw the discard amount according to institutions protocol (usually 3 to 6 cc) but at least 1.5 times the internal catheter volume.

Syringe-collection method: A 10-cc syringe is commonly used when drawing a blood sample from a CVC. However, if drawing a sample is difficult, use a 5-cc syringe or smaller. When drawing the blood specimen, use practices that reduce trauma to the blood cells, such as using larger needles (20 gauge or larger), having patience when drawing laboratory specimens, and not pulling the plunger way back in an effort to hurry the withdrawal process. There is a very specific order for filling specimen tubes. Improper order can result in contamination of the sample with inappropriate additives. Laboratory tubes are color-coded. The NCCLS recommends that, when using a syringe, tubes with anticoagulants are filled first. This method reduces the potential for blood clotting in the syringe. The order for filling laboratory tubes using the syringe method is as follows:

1. Citrate tubes (light blue top)
2. Heparin tubes (green top)
3. EDTA (ethylenediaminetetraacetic acid) tubes (lavender top)
4. Oxalate and sodium fluoride tubes (gray top)
5. Gel separator tubes and clot activator tubes (speckled or mottled top)
6. Nonadditive or serum tubes (red top)

Vacutainer method: The vacuum in the tubes is high, and a rapid draw through a small-lumen catheter (e.g., a Broviac®, 24-gauge PICC) can traumatize red blood cells. After flushing, attach the vacutainer to the CVC and push on a red top tube. Fill the red top tube completely. This tube is the discard tube. Label and discard. Collect tubes that form a clot first (opposite of syringe-collection method). This action prevents the vacutainer spike from being contaminated with additives. The order for filling laboratory tubes using the vacutainer method is as follows:

1. Nonadditive tubes (red top)
2. Citrate tubes (light blue top)
3. Heparin tubes (green top)
4. EDTA tubes (lavender top)
5. Gel separator tubes and clot activator tubes (speckled or mottled top)
6. Other

Coagulation studies, as a general rule, should not be drawn through the CVC. However, if the CVC must be used to collect the specimen, the machines in the laboratory can be recalibrated for accurate results. This procedure will result in additional time and cost and should be done as a last option.

Amount of blood in each tube: Overfilling or underfilling tubes should be avoided. With tubes containing additives, the correct amount of blood is essential to maintain the additive-to-blood ratio necessary for reliable results. When blue tubes are underfilled, the coagulation results are prolonged. When lavender tubes are underfilled, the cell counts and hematocrit results may be low. If a tube is overfilled, it can cause the stopper to dislodge, leading to blood contamination. When attaching the syringe to the tube, blood will be drawn into the tube automatically. When the blood stops moving into the tube, remove the syringe and begin filling the next tube until all the specimens have been collected.

Immediately after filling, gently rock tubes containing additives (purple, blue, green) a minimum of 8 to 10 times. This action will ensure the proper mixing of the additives with the blood. Do not rock tubes that do not contain additives (red stopper tubes). Do not shake any tube. Label tubes immediately after drawing the specimen at the patient's bedside according to institution protocol. Follow the institution's policy for transporting to laboratory.

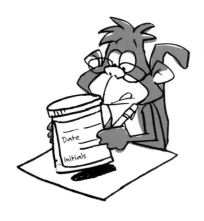

⚠ Patient's treatment is partially based on laboratory test results; thus improper labeling can result in undertreatment or overtreatment. Deaths have occurred because blood tubes were not labeled properly with the correct patient's identification. Label blood tubes at the patient's bedside.

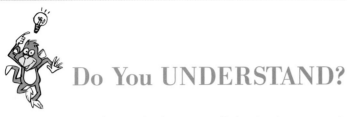

Do You UNDERSTAND?

DIRECTIONS: **Place a check next to all the disadvantages of using the syringe-collection method of collecting blood from a CVC for purposes of laboratory analysis.**

1. a. _____ Increased potential for blood exposure
   b. _____ Potential for overfilling tubes
   c. _____ Syringe automatically fills
   d. _____ Even and consistent pressure on vein
   e. _____ Need to change syringes while holding onto vacutainer
   f. _____ Requires transferring blood specimen to the tube

DIRECTIONS: **Choose the one correct answer in the parentheses for each statement.**

2. If a lavender tube is underfilled, the hematocrit results will be falsely _____. *(low* or *high)*
3. If blue tubes for coagulation studies are underfilled, the results will be _____. *(prolonged* or *shortened)*
4. Shaking a laboratory tube will cause red blood cell _____. *(overproduction* or *hemolysis)*

What IS Removal of a Central Venous Catheter?

All CVCs should be removed (i.e., taken out of the patient's body) when they are no longer indicated. If there is any question of loss of catheter integrity, the catheter is removed immediately. Improper removal technique can result in catheter damage, fracture, or both.

Answers: 1. a, b, f; 2. low; 3. prolonged; 4. hemolysis.

What You NEED TO KNOW

Specially trained nurses can remove PICCs and nontunneled CVCs (according to institution protocol). Physicians remove tunneled catheters, as well as implanted and Swan-Ganz catheters. Consideration should be given to factors that may induce resistance to removal, including venous spasm, phlebitis (PICCs, arm ports), thrombosis, fibrin formation, or knotting of the catheter. When thrombosis is suspected, removal should *not* be attempted until the physician has investigated and tests have been performed for confirmation of size and location of the thrombosis. Air embolism (sudden obstruction of a blood vessel by a bolus of air that has entered the circulatory system) is most often associated with STCVC removal. The STCVC track may remain open for a very brief moment.

 A CVC track formed with a 14-gauge catheter can transmit about 200 ml of air in 1 second, which is enough to form an air embolism.

What You DO

STCVC: Removal requires special knowledge to minimize the potential for air embolism, prevent catheter damage, and to ensure hemostasis of the insertion site. Equipment necessary for removal includes suture removal kit (if sutures are present), dressing change kit, sterile gauze, and petroleum-based ointment or Vaseline gauze. The nurse must wash hands and put on nonsterile gloves before removal of old dressing. As with all procedures, first explain the procedure to the patient and allow time for questions and answers.

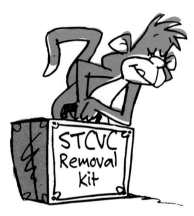

1. Open suture removal kit. Open dressing change kit.
2. Open sterile gauze and drop into dressing change kit.
3. Apply a bleb of petroleum-based ointment (according to the Infusion Nursing Society [INS], such as Vaseline or antimicrobial ointment) to the center of the dressing.
4. Position the patient in the supine position.
5. Clamp all pigtails and remove the dressing.
6. Apply sterile gloves and clean the site (see dressing change).
7. Remove sutures.
8. With nondominant hand, hold the gauze over the site.
9. Have the patient perform a Valsalva maneuver (hold breath and bear down) in medically appropriate patients.

10. With dominant hand, pull the CVC out parallel to the skin in one, even motion.

11. As soon as the tip of the catheter clears the exit site, immediately cover the insertion site with the gauze, making sure the petroleum-based ointment covers the insertion site. The petroleum-based ointment seals the insertion site, preventing air entry.

12. If culturing the tip, drop the catheter into the sterile dressing change kit to prevent any contamination of the catheter.

13. Hold pressure over site for 5 minutes or longer to ensure hemostasis.

14. Cover the gauze with tape or transparent dressing, forming an occlusive dressing to ensure hemostasis.

15. Inspect the catheter tip for integrity.

16. Have the patient remain lying down for 30 minutes.

17. Leave the dressing in place for 12 to 24 hours.

18. Document appearance of insertion site, the integrity of the catheter, and patient response.

> **Do not have a cardiac patient perform the Valsalva maneuver because bradycardia may result.**

> **It is important not to apply firm pressure or forceful rubbing of the neck over the carotid artery. Messaging the insertion site after CVC removal from an internal jugular can dislodge atherosclerotic plaque or thrombus in the carotid artery, which may cause a stroke. Carotid stimulation can also cause bradycardia.**

Removal: Removal requires special knowledge to minimize the potential for venous spasm and prevent catheter damage. When removing a PICC, manipulation of the smooth muscle can be stimulated, causing a venous spasm. Phlebitis can increase the occurrence of venous spasm by increasing the vein's response to stimulation. To minimize venous spasm, apply a warm compress to the upper arm about 20 minutes before the removal process to enhance venous dilatation and blood flow around the catheter and to minimize innervating the smooth muscles. It may be helpful to leave the compress in place for the duration of the removal procedure. To minimize potential damage to the catheter, the catheter should be grasped at the insertion site and slowly pulled out parallel to the skin in 1-inch segments. Minimal pressure should be exerted, and the catheter should not be stretched. The procedure should be stopped if the patient verbalizes the presence of sharp pain or other sensations along the catheter tract or if any resistance is felt during removal. Forceful removal may result in significant trauma to the vein wall that may cause additional thrombus formation and possibly vein perforation. Radiologic studies may be indicated to determine the status of the catheter before further removal attempts are made. Catheters that are coated with a fibrin sheath or are attached to the vein wall secondary to thrombus formation may have to be surgically removed. Once the PICC is completely removed, apply the gauze to the puncture site and apply light pressure until homeostasis is achieved and then apply tape. Observe the tip of the catheter for integrity and measure the total length. Compare this measurement with the originally documented length. If a discrepancy

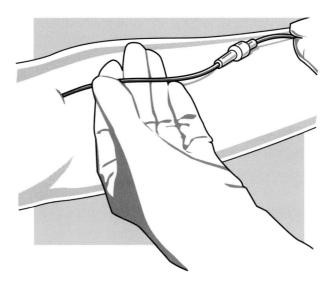

between insertion length and removal length is identified, lightly apply a tourniquet to the upper arm and notify the physician immediately. Document per the institution's protocol, including site appearance, catheter length and integrity, and all patient comments.

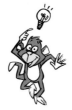

Do You UNDERSTAND?

DIRECTIONS: **Choose the one correct answer in parentheses for each statement.**

1. A CVC should be removed from the patient's body with the CVC being _____ to the patient's skin. *(parallel* or *perpendicular)*

2. Pressure over the cephalic site of a removed CVC should last for at least _____ minutes. *(5* or *25)*

3. Before removing a PICC, the nurse should place a _____ compress over the PICC site to enhance venous dilatation. *(warm* or *cold)*

4. _____ embolism is most often associated with nontunneled CVC removal. *(Fat* or *Air)*

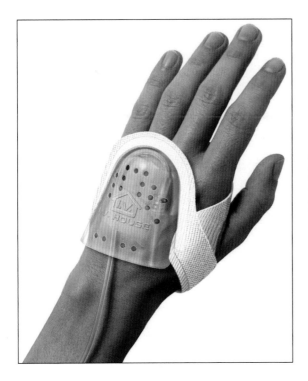

PLATE 1. **Catheter protection.** A plastic dome protects the catheter insertion site and stress prevention loop, minimizing the likelihood of catheter dislodgment.

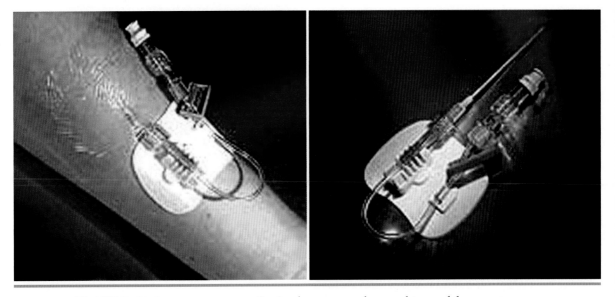

PLATE 2. **Catheter securement.** StatLock secures catheter tubing and forms a stress prevention loop, making the use of tape unnecessary to secure the tubing.

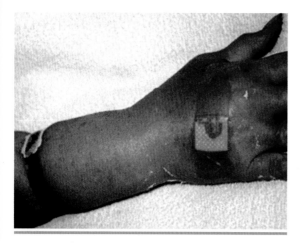

PLATE 3. **Infiltration.** Infiltration has caused tissue swelling.

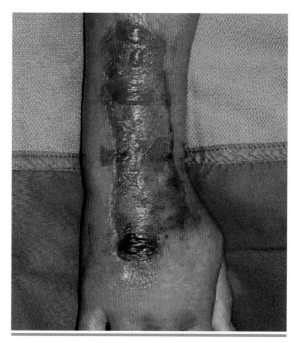

PLATE 4. **Mild extravasation.** Mild extravasation includes blistering and swelling.

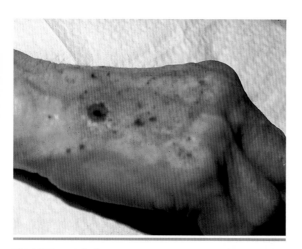

PLATE 5. **Moderate extravasation.** Moderate extravasation includes ulcer formation.

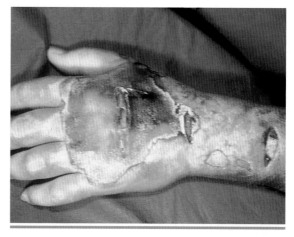

PLATE 6. **Severe extravasation.** Tissue sloughing is a result of severe extravasation.

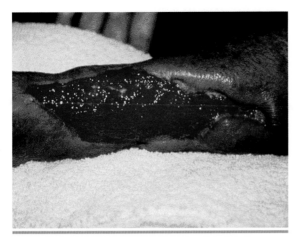

PLATE 7. **Extreme extravasation.** Extreme extravasation includes extensive tissue sloughing and will require plastic surgery to remedy.

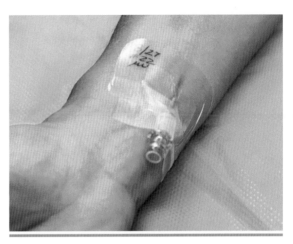

PLATE 8. **Mechanical phlebitis.** A red streak over the catheter track is a sign of mechanical phlebitis.

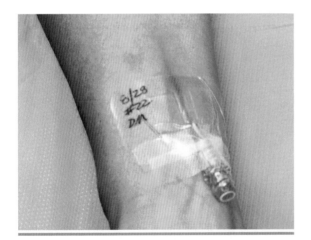

PLATE 9. **Chemical phlebitis.** A red streak over the vein track above the catheter tip indicates chemical phlebitis.

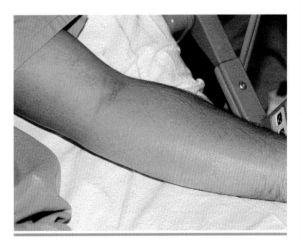

PLATE 10. **Severe chemical phlebitis.** A generalized, extreme inflammation of the venous tree indicates severe chemical phlebitis.

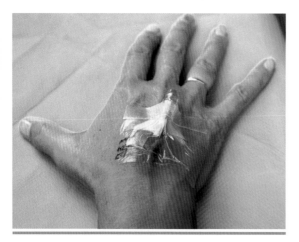

PLATE 11. **Hematoma.** Hematoma has occurred at the catheter insertion site.

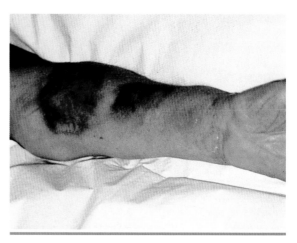

PLATE 12. **Hematoma.** Severe hematoma has occurred at the time of catheter removal.

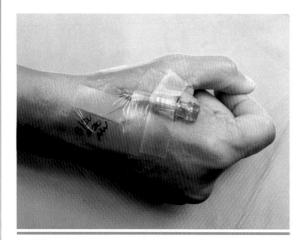

PLATE 13. **Local site infection.** Redness and swelling localized at the insertion site indicate local site infection.

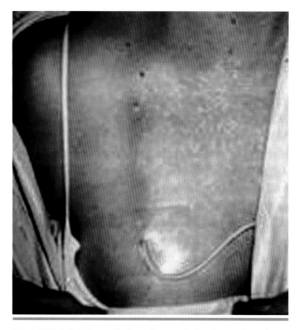

PLATE 14. **Tunneled catheter infection.** A reddened area anywhere along the catheter tunnel may indicate a tunneled catheter infection.

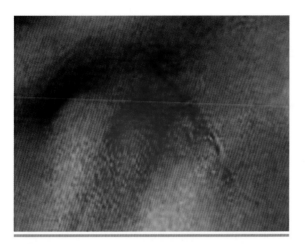

PLATE 15. **Port pocket infection.** A reddened area over the port pocket may indicate infection.

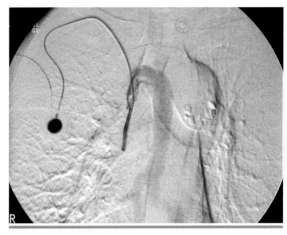

PLATE 16. **Fibrin sheath with retrograde flow.** In a dye study of clot characteristics, retrograde flow is shown when the dye is located above the catheter tip.

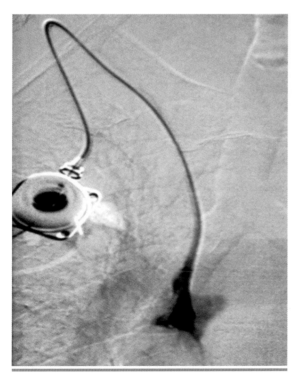

PLATE 17. **Catheter pinch off.** A pinched-off catheter shows the catheter compressed between the clavicle and first rib.

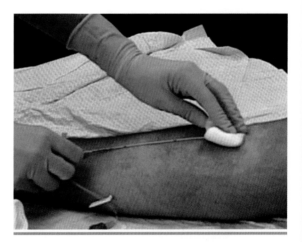

PLATE 18: **Catheter shearing and fracture.** Excessive pulling with PICC removal can result in catheter shearing and fracture.

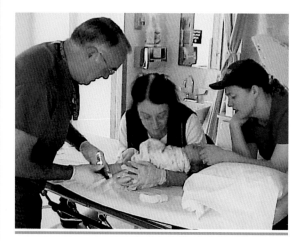

PLATE 19. **Child holder.** An individual should hold the child to assist in catheter insertion. The only appendage free should be the one in which the IV catheter is inserted.

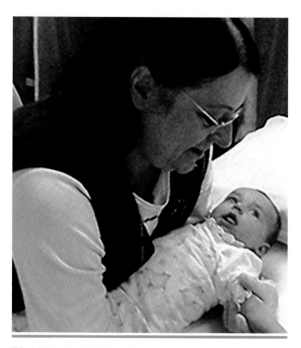

PLATE 20. **Child holder holding swaddled infant.** The individual holding a swaddled infant in preparation for IV catheter insertion should support and elevate the infant's head. This method helps keep the infant calm and may prevent a stressed infant from vomiting, a common occurrence.

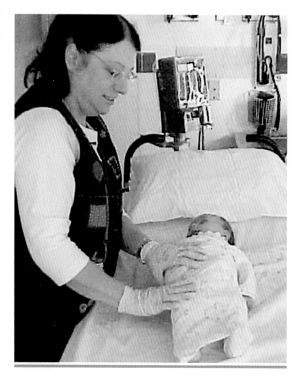

PLATE 21. **Infant swaddled in a blanket.** Swaddling an infant makes it easy for the individual holding the child to control and minimize infant movement during IV catheter insertion.

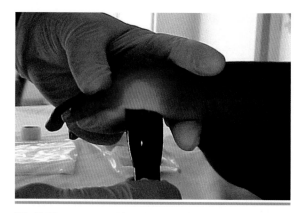

PLATE 22. **Transillumination of veins using a flashlight.** Illuminating a child's veins with a light source is a nonthreatening approach to vein visualization. Children are usually interested in the procedure. The proper positioning of light is needed to visualize the venous network.

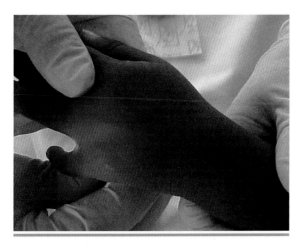

PLATE 23. **Vein visualization.** A significant amount of time should be spent visualizing a child's venous network to select the best vein for IV catheter insertion.

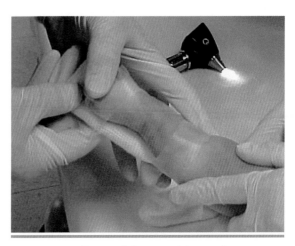

PLATE 24. **Vein stabilization.** Taping the arm to a board will give support to the hand or arm, enabling traction to be applied to the vein chosen as the IV catheter insertion site.

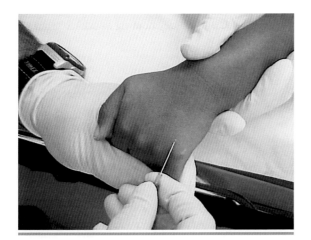

PLATE 25. **Vein stabilization.** Bending the fingers down toward the inner arm will make the hand more stable, enabling sufficient traction to be applied to the vein chosen as the IV catheter insertion site.

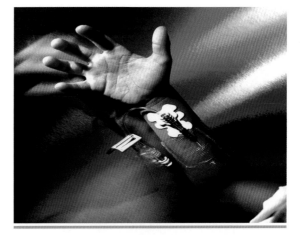

PLATE 26. **Catheter stabilization.** Catheter stabilization and connection padding minimize the possibility of catheter dislodgment and protect the skin.

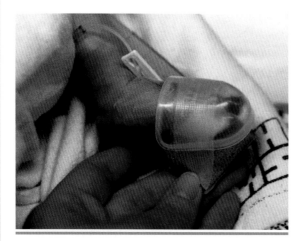

PLATE 27. Catheter stabilization. Insertion site protection stabilizes the catheter and minimizes the potential that even the smallest infant may "rub out" the catheter.

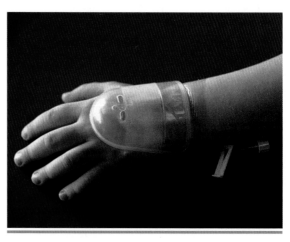

PLATE 28. Insertion site protection. Insertion site protection minimizes catheter dislodgment and insertion site trauma.

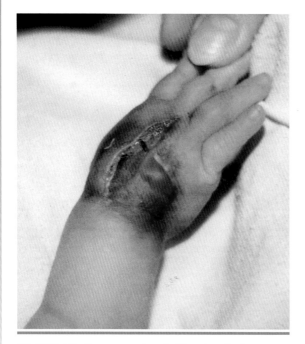

PLATE 29. Extravasation. Infiltration is the most common pediatric IV complication. Particular attention must be given to the child receiving vesicant medications.

Insert illustration credits

Plates 1, 27, and 28: Courtesy IV House, St. Louis, Mo.

Plates 2, 19, 20, 21, 22, 23, 24, 25, 26: Courtesy Venetec International, San Diego, Calif.

Plates 5, 6, 8, 9, 10, 11, 13, 14, and 29: Courtesy Professional Learning Systems, Inc., Atlanta, Ga.

Plates 15, 16, and 17: Courtesy Judy Peckel, RN, OCN.

Plate 18: Courtesy PICC Excellence, Inc., Oak Park, Fla.

Central Venous Catheter Complications

Top Bananas: Chapter 5 Overview

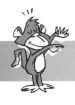

What IS a Central Venous Catheter Complication?

A central venous catheter (CVC) complication is a problem that results from having a CVC in place. Risk increases from peripheral access to central venous access. Complications or problems associated with CVCs are more

127

serious than are those with peripheral lines, requiring greater understanding to identify and treat the problems as they occur. By far, the most effective way to manage complications with CVCs is to prevent them from happening. A comprehensive understanding of the possible complications with central venous devices is vital to optimal management. It is important to be aware of all complications that can occur, to be able to identify problems early before they become more serious, to know what actions to take when they do occur, and to implement prevention methods whenever possible.

 ## What You NEED TO KNOW

 TAKE HOME POINTS

Be aware that **arrhythmia,** an irregular change in the heart beat, and **dysrhythmia,** an irregular change of the heart rhythm, are terms that are often used interchangeably in the clinical setting.

Complications that occur with CVCs can be localized or systemic in nature. These complications include:

- Infection, local or systemic (sepsis)
- Venous thrombosis
- Phlebitis
- Arrhythmias
- Pneumothorax (air) and hemothorax (blood)
- Mast cell activation syndrome and allergic reactions
- Circulatory overload and pulmonary edema
- Hemorrhage
- Emboli

Catheter events are problems that happen to the catheter. These events can occur upon insertion, as a result of accidents, failure to follow flushing protocols or other actions of the medical professional. Catheter events include:

- Occlusion
- Catheter damage and breakage
- Malpositioning and migration
- Pinch-off syndrome

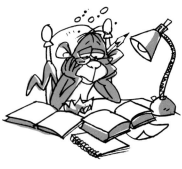 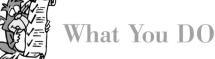 ## What You DO

Prevention: Many complications can be prevented through understanding on the part of the nurse, medical team, and through patient education. Education is a primary tool to prevent complications, allowing the clinician to anticipate problems and avoid the development of some complications. Certain CVCs are more prone to specific complications (e.g., phlebitis with peripherally inserted central catheters [PICCs], sepsis with nontunneled CVCs). Infection control, the intravenous (IV) team, risk management, or the PICC team can tell the nurse the most frequently occurring complications within his or her institution, based on CVC outcome monitoring.

Assessment: Early identification of complications means the ability to pick up early symptoms, warnings, and clues to impending problems before they become serious or life threatening.

Early symptoms are specific to the complication but may include, restlessness, anxiety, fever, pain, swelling, redness, inability to flush, changes in the device position, or electrocardiogram (ECG) changes. Collaboration among health care providers with free communication is beneficial to the patient and aids in the early identification of complications, resulting in subsequent action.

Treatment: Once a complication has been identified, effort is needed to stabilize the complication and avoid worsening of the problem. For example, if the catheter has broken, a clamp needs to be applied to avoid air being drawn into the body that may result in air emboli. The physician should be made aware of any complications associated with CVCs. What the nurse should do with CVCs depends on the specific complication.

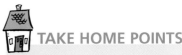

TAKE HOME POINTS

- It is important to be aware of all potential complications associated with CVCs.
- Know the most frequent complications for the institution to more easily detect them early and avoid the development of more serious problems.
- Prevent complications by acting on clues early, collaborating with other clinicians, and educating the patient and staff of potential hazards.

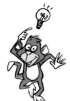

Do You UNDERSTAND?

DIRECTIONS: **Match the subject from Column A with the definition from Column B.**

Column A

1. _____ Complication
2. _____ Methods to deal with complications
3. _____ Prevention

Column B

a. Detect potential problems early
b. Educate staff and patients on warning signs
c. A problem that develops

Answers: 1. c; 2. b; 3. a.

DIRECTIONS: **Find and circle the following words.**

air	catheter	infection	occlusions
arrhythmia	damage	malpositioning	pneumothorax
breakage	emboli	migration	phlebitis

T	M	O	N	V	I	S	Z	Z	Y	A	T	V	K
X	A	R	O	H	T	O	M	U	E	N	P	X	P
D	L	F	I	W	Y	F	O	D	P	C	T	D	A
S	P	C	T	T	O	E	U	P	L	K	Q	R	O
D	O	C	C	L	U	S	I	O	N	S	R	X	U
R	S	O	E	S	M	H	Q	V	N	H	O	F	M
N	I	U	F	B	F	E	Q	T	Y	H	O	S	K
V	T	A	N	O	M	R	E	T	E	H	T	A	C
S	I	T	I	B	E	L	H	P	F	Q	G	E	V
Q	O	A	O	R	B	M	E	Y	N	P	R	M	Y
C	N	L	V	E	I	D	Z	M	Q	D	V	U	J
M	I	G	R	A	T	I	O	N	C	Q	L	K	F
A	N	K	M	K	M	Y	Q	E	N	R	Y	P	I
E	G	A	M	A	D	J	A	I	L	H	Q	Q	K
Y	E	X	K	G	Z	J	J	Y	R	L	A	J	H
G	Y	X	C	E	V	O	M	J	C	M	P	T	C

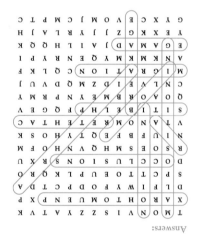

Answers:

What IS a Central Venous Catheter Infection?

An *infection* is the presence of pathogenic organisms that reproduce and multiply in a quantity sufficient to cause symptoms or disease. According to the Centers for Disease Control and Prevention (CDC), the presence of a CVC is a risk factor for infection. Infections associated with CVCs can be either **local** (bacterial growth on the skin surrounding the CVC) or **systemic** (throughout the body). Infections are the most serious complication that can result from the presence and use of a CVC as a result of the morbidity involved (i.e., of/or related to illness, the ability to cause a person to be sick). As a result of the serious risk associated with CVC-related infection, early identification of symptoms can help limit the spread of the infection. An example is a local infection; if quickly identified and treated, it will not become a systemic infection.

What You NEED TO KNOW

Symptoms that reflect an infectious process are the following:
- Fever
- Heart rate increase
- Changes in respiration rate or pattern
- Redness, swelling, heat at the site, or any combination
- Gastrointestinal symptoms (e.g., diarrhea, vomiting, pain)
- Central nervous system involvement (e.g., dizziness, blurred vision)
- Fatigue
- Drainage, pus, or serosanquinous fluid around the device or insertion site

TAKE HOME POINTS

The presence of drainage requires an immediate order for insertion site and CVC culture. Common sources of catheter contamination are the following:
- Hands of the medical personnel
- Patient's skin microflora
- Hub colonization of bacteria
- Contamination on CVC insertion
- Contaminated infusate
- Bacteria transported by the patient's blood (**hematogenous spread**)

Sources of Catheter Contamination

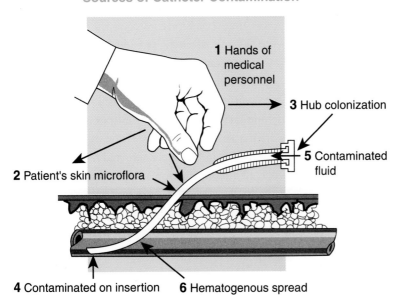

1 Hands of medical personnel

3 Hub colonization

5 Contaminated fluid

2 Patient's skin microflora

4 Contaminated on insertion

6 Hematogenous spread

Patients who are immunocompromised, infants, and older adults may have delayed or varied symptoms, including but not limited to:

- Temperature intolerance
- Reduced heart rate (bradycardia)
- Loss of appetite
- Fatigue

What You DO

Preventation: Preventative measures for CVC infections include the following:

- Use of meticulous sterile technique and preparation with the insertion of any CVC
- Care and maintenance that includes changing tubing and caps at regular policy intervals and swabbing IV access ports with alcohol or povidone iodine, using friction before any access
- Use of sterile caps
- Meticulous dressing management (see Chapter 4)
- Insertion of CVC—impregnated or coated-antiseptic or coated-antimicrobial catheters in patients at risk for infection, such as those who are receiving total parenteral nutrition (TPN), are neutropenic, and are in the intensive care unit, as well as those whose catheter remains in place more than 4 days (according to the CDC)
- Reading journal articles and research, attending product in-services, and industrial showcase at conventions to keep informed of new products designed to prevent complications

Assessment: CVCs presenting with redness and swelling at the insertion site with no other symptoms may have a local site infection (see color plates 14 and 15). It is necessary to rule out systemic infection by looking for other symptoms, such as fever, changes in blood pressure and heart rate, or other symptoms that may indicate a more widespread infection. Systemic infections most commonly require the CVC to be removed with the catheter tip cut off and sent to the lab for culture and sensitivity (C & S) tests (see Chapter 4).

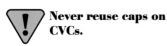

Never reuse caps on CVCs.

www.ons.org
(Oncology Nursing Society)
www.ins1.org
(Infusion Nursing Society)
www.navannet.org
(National Association of Venous Access Networks)

Treatment: Local treatment focuses on the type and extent of the infection. Some local infections can be easily treated with topical antibiotics; other local infections require removal of the CVC. Treatment of a systemic infection associated with a CVC follows a common pattern:

1. Obtain multiple culture results to identify an organism.
2. Administer organism-specific antibiotics based on C & S results.
3. Reinsert the CVC, if necessary. The CDC recommends using prophylactic antibiotic lock solution in treating a patient with a long-term catheter or port who has a history of multiple systemic infections, despite optimal aseptic technique.

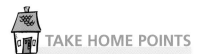

TAKE HOME POINTS

Blood cultures and site cultures are taken whenever an infection is suspected. Catheter tip cultures are taken with the removal of any CVC associated with infection.

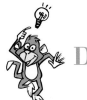

Do You UNDERSTAND?

DIRECTIONS: Unscramble each of the symptoms of infection.

1. _____ *(ferve)*

2. _____ *(reessdn)*

3. _____ *(peeruratmet hegcan)*

4. _____ *(arhte raet cirneesa)*

5. _____ *(denraiag)*

6. _____ *(ilwlesng)*

7. _____ *(sepnirtaior segncha)*

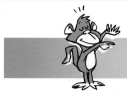

What IS Venous Thrombosis?

Venous thrombosis is an accumulation of clotted blood within a vein caused by (1) injury, irritation, or diseased changes (plaque, atherosclerosis), causing alteration of the vein wall; (2) stasis of blood, obstruction, or change in blood flow from a catheter, all within a vein; or (3) aggregation of blood resulting from a hypercoaguable state.

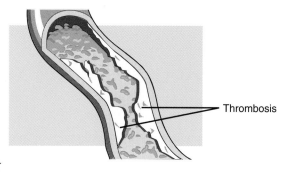

Thrombosis

What You NEED TO KNOW

Triad of Virchow

These three causative factors are called the *triad of Virchow,* named after the eighteenth century physician who studied coagulation of blood. Understanding causation of thrombosis, symptoms, and methods of prevention will help in managing patients with CVCs, resulting in better outcomes.

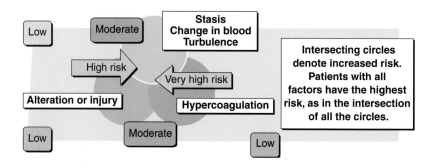

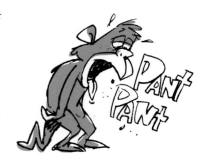

The result of untreated thrombosis is inhibition and eventual cessation of blood flow, potential for permanent injury to the vein wall, loss of function of a central venous device, pain to the patient with the development of collateral vessels, shortness of breath if the vessel affected restricts blood flow to the heart as in superior vena cava (SVC) syndrome, swelling in the tissues surrounding the developing thrombosis, and the potential for pieces to break off and result in pulmonary emboli.

CVCs carry a risk of venous thrombosis because of their presence in a vessel. Catheters cause injury on insertion, can irritate vein walls, and change the flow of blood in a vein, resulting in points of stasis. Injury, irritation, and blood stasis can all precipitate clot development. Insertion of a needle through the skin results in injury that leads to clot formation. If other factors such as irritation, lack of blood flow, or high platelet levels are present, the clot may continue to grow and develop into a more serious thrombus. Fibrinolysis is a constant process in the body; clots are broken down naturally every minute of every day. The goal is to keep clot-forming factors at a minimum, prevent occlusive thrombi, and thus avoid detrimental outcomes.

Characteristics of Clots

Blood clots associated with CVCs have different characteristics based on the cause of clot propagation and the body's response. Fibrin covers a catheter within minutes of insertion as a natural body response to foreign matter. Clot formation around a catheter varies and includes:

- Inside the catheter lumen (intraluminal thrombus)
- At the tip of the catheter (fibrin tail)

Inside Catheter Lumen

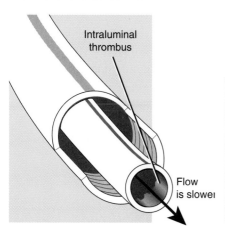

Intraluminal thrombus

Flow is slower

Catheter Tip

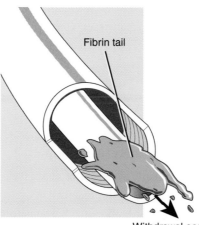

Fibrin tail

Withdrawal occlusion

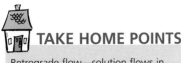

TAKE HOME POINTS

Retrograde flow—solution flows in the space between the fibrin sheath and the external catheter wall (see color plate 16).

Catheter (External Wall)

Fibrin sheath

Retrograde flow

Vein Wall

Vein wall

Mural thrombus

Flow slows as external pressure on outside of catheter increases

- Attaches to external wall of catheter (fibrin sheath)
- Attaches to the vein wall (mural thrombus) and exerts pressure on the outside of the catheter

The body responds to clot development by sending clot busters (**fibrinolytics**) to the site, which are natural enzymes designed to dissolve the clot. The body uses some of these same enzymes, primarily in recombinant forms, also known as thrombolytics, to dissolve clotted catheters.

Risk Factors

Risk factors for thrombosis include high platelet levels, advanced age, smoking, pregnancy, oral contraceptive use, lung cancer, gynecologic malignancies, sickle cell anemia, deficiency of anticoagulant factors, multitrauma, surgery, diabetes, previous history of deep venous thrombosis, and chronic obstructive pulmonary disease, to name a few. Other risk factors include catheters placed via the left subclavian vein, malpositioning of the catheter, catheter tip location in the subclavian vein rather than in the SVC, intrathoracic tumor, and engorgement of the upper trunk vessels, resulting from compression of the SVC by an extrinsic mass.

Symptoms of Thrombosis

An early symptom of clot development is persistent withdrawal occlusion (PWO), or the inability to aspirate blood from a CVC. The CVC may or may not flush easily; but something is preventing withdrawal of blood, usu-

TAKE HOME POINTS

Symptoms of pain, leakage at the insertion site, swelling, and inability to aspirate blood are all signs of thrombosis.

ally a clot. PWO is common with implanted ports, valved catheters, and PICCs. Another sign of thrombus development includes leaking at the insertion site, which occurs because the fluid is unable to flow out of the catheter and flows backward instead. When a large sleevelike thrombus develops around a catheter, the fluid may be able to flow out the end of the catheter. However, instead of flowing into the bloodstream, the fluid flows between the thrombus sleeve and the outer wall of the catheter back toward the insertion site. Symptoms of infiltration or extravasation can occur near the insertion site with swelling, redness, and potential sloughing of skin (with vesicants; see Chapter 3). The larger a thrombus is, the greater the risk is of pieces breaking off and becoming emboli within the body. Deep vein thrombosis (DVT) is a condition in which the thrombus occludes a large, vital vein, such as the subclavian vein or the SVC. Symptoms of DVT are more serious, more pronounced, and include sudden pain, swelling that develops rapidly, and numbness or tingling in the extremity. The size of a clot involved in DVT continues to increase. When the thrombosis obstructs the vein, blood pools and sticks together, resulting in an ever-expanding clot. Think of a dam in a stream: sticks and dirt collect behind it making the obstruction bigger; water pushes up against it, rising higher on the banks. The clot acts as the dam, and the IV fluid and blood act as the water. The body responds with the development of collateral veins to go around the clot (dam), and the venous stasis causes swelling as fluid leaks out of the vein into the tissue. DVT must be resolved quickly.

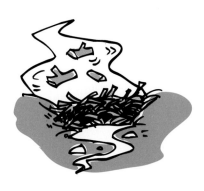

 # What You DO

Assessment: It is important to identify patients who are at risk for thrombosis so that close, ongoing assessment can be done. Notify the physician of the potential thrombosis or clot, and discuss the options. Some physicians order low-dose oral anticoagulants for high-risk patients. Observation for thrombosis development includes being alert to primary symptoms of pain, swelling, and tingling. These symptoms can be vague, generalized, or focused, near the CVC or elsewhere.

Signs and symptoms of thrombosis development are sometimes vague, difficult to pinpoint, and may appear to be other types of complications. Symptoms may not be present as a thrombus is developing, occurring only after the thrombosis is large enough to cause obstruction of blood flow.

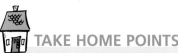 TAKE HOME POINTS

Only 5% of subclavian vein thromboses are symptomatic as a result of collateral circulation development.

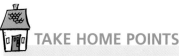 TAKE HOME POINTS

Do not dismiss symptoms; be vigilant in identifying their causes.

Treatment: Treatment of thrombosis depends on the extent of the symptoms and the size of the clot. Some physicians will refer the patient with a potential thrombosis directly to radiology. Definite diagnosis of a thrombosis is made in radiology through a venogram or cathetergram. Ultrasound or sonogram is also used to identify clot formation; but these are not as specific as are the previously mentioned tests and may miss small clots in or around the catheter. If a thrombosis is identified, the physician will determine the thrombolytic protocol based on size of the clot. Using a thrombolytic early with PWO may reduce the risk of subsequent clot formation. Other options are a brushing technique for removal of clots within a catheter or surgical removal of the clot, as in a thrombectomy.

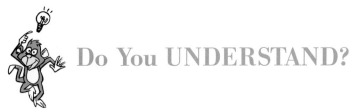

Do You UNDERSTAND?

DIRECTIONS: **Unscramble the letters to form the predisposing conditions for thrombosis.**

MONKISG ☐☐☐☐☐☐☐

PENGAYCRN ☐☐☐☐☐☐☐☐☐

BIHRT CNTOOLR PSLIL ☐☐☐☐☐ ☐☐☐☐☐☐☐ ☐☐☐☐☐

TOILYIMBMI ☐☐☐☐☐☐☐☐☐☐

CRNACE ☐☐☐☐☐☐

TUAMAR ☐☐☐☐☐☐

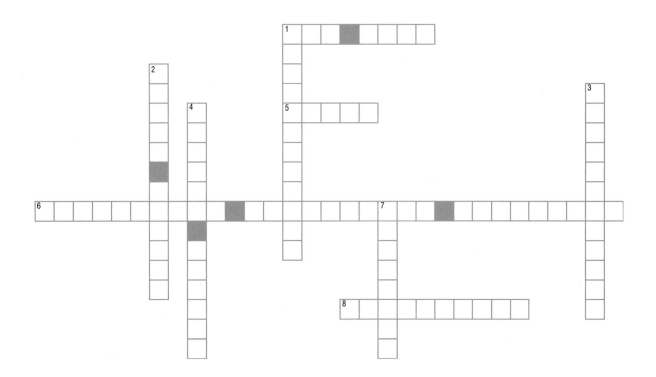

DIRECTIONS: **Complete the above crossword puzzle using the following clues.**

Across

1. Red blood cells and fibrin that attach to a catheter tip and hang down. (*two words*)
5. A thrombus that attaches to a vein wall and catheter.
6. Able to flush but not aspirate blood (*three words*)
8. Development of a clot within a vessel, many of which are asymptomatic

Down

1. Type of medication used to treat clotted blood or fibrin buildup
2. Cause of thrombosis associated with blood flow (*two words*)
3. Clot buster
4. Forms on outside of catheter
7. Oral medication used to prevent clot development or growth

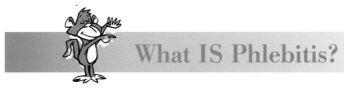

What IS Phlebitis?

Phlebitis is the inflammation of the vein wall.

What You NEED TO KNOW

Phlebitis is the most common complication associated with PICCs (5% of cases after insertion). Phlebitis can be caused by powder from gloves, irritating medications or solutions, threading too fast, rigid catheters, large-gauge catheters (restricts blood flow), or from bacterial contamination. Sterile phlebitis may occur within the first 24 to 48 hours after insertion as a direct response to the foreign material in the body. Catheter tips that are placed in vessels other than the SVC place the person at risk for chemical phlebitis and thrombosis (for more information, see Chapter 3).

What You DO

Prevention: See Chapter 4, "PICC Insertion, What You Do."

Treatment: Treatment for phlebitis is based on a prescription for continuous warm compress application to the extremity with the PICC at the first sign of pain or swelling. If no improvement or worsening occurs within 24 to 48 hours, the line will need to be removed based on a physician order. Because phlebitis may be a precursor to thrombosis and infection, the catheter is removed when there is no response to treatment (see Chapter 4, "PICC Removal").

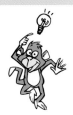

Do You UNDERSTAND?

DIRECTIONS: **In the spaces provided, identify the causes of phlebitis with a "C" and the symptoms of phlebitis with an "S."**

1. _____ Foreign material in body
2. _____ Swelling
3. _____ Inflammation along the catheter line
4. _____ Too small a vein for blood flow around catheter
5. _____ Wrong terminal tip location
6. _____ Rigid catheter
7. _____ Redness
8. _____ Powder on gloves
9. _____ Medication or chemical irritation
10. _____ Pain

What IS an Arrhythmia Associated with Central Venous Devices?

An arrhythmia, or irregular heartbeat, is present with CVC insertion when the device is advanced into the heart, causing stimulation of the atrioventricular (AV) or sinoatrial (SA) nodes.

What You NEED TO KNOW

Symptoms of an arrhythmia include a feeling of heaviness, difficulty breathing, or extreme anxiety. Resolution is based on identification of the arrhythmia and retraction of the CVC to proper placement. If a patient begins complaining of a feeling of fullness in the head, difficulty breathing,

Answers: 1. C; 2. S; 3. S; 4. C; 5. C; 6. C; 7. S; 8. C; 9. C; 10. S.

and something lying on the chest, the CVC has gone into the right atrium too deeply; pull it back. The cause of arrhythmias is stimulation of the AV or SA node in the heart wall. X-ray confirmation can identify asymptomatic deep insertions with posteroanterior (PA) and lateral films.

What You DO

Retraction of the catheter is done first; pulling back the catheter to the level that the radiologist specifies will usually resolve the arrhythmia. Prevention focuses on accurate measurement for proper catheter placement, clear prompt x-rays for placement, and the avoidance of intentional deep insertions.

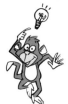

Do You UNDERSTAND?

DIRECTIONS: **In the spaces provided, identify the statements that are** *true* **with a "T" and those that are** *false* **with an "F."**

1. _____ Prevention focuses on accurate measurement for proper catheter placement.
2. _____ Prevention focuses on clear prompt x-rays for placement.
3. _____ Prevention focuses on the avoidance of intentional deep insertions.
4. _____ When a patient states they feel a heaviness in their chest during catheter advancement, the catheter is in the correct location.
5. _____ The cause of arrhythmias is stimulation of the AV or SA node in the heart wall.

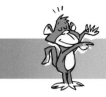

What IS Air Emboli Associated with a CVC?

Air embolism is the sudden obstruction of a blood vessel by a bolus of air that has entered the circulatory system.

What You NEED TO KNOW

When an air embolus enters the heart, it acts as a mechanical obstruction in the right ventricle, preventing blood flow. The pulmonary artery oxygen is denied to the lungs. Factors that affect the relative risk of an air emboli include size of the CVC, distance of the CVC to the heart, position of access above or below the heart, length of time the access site is open to air, and the activity of the patient. Air emboli can occur on insertion of a CVC, when using the CVC, when tubing connections or injection caps are left open to air, or at the time of CVC removal. Although air emboli can occur with any CVC (given the right conditions), it is most often associated with nontunneled, CVC removal. The short track present when a short-term multilumen central catheter is removed may stay open for a brief moment. A CVC track formed with a 14-gauge catheter can transmit about 200 ml of air in 1 second.

The mortality of the patient who is experiencing air emboli is based on the amount of air and rate at which the air enters the body, as well as the promptness of the treatment.

Symptoms of air emboli include the following:
- Anxiety
- Light-headedness
- Confusion
- Shortness of breath
- Air hunger
- Pallor
- Increased heart rate (tachycardia)
- Decreased blood pressure (hypotension)
- Possible cyanosis

What You DO

Prevention: Prime all tubing before use. Change solutions before they are completely dry. Attach piggyback medications to the highest infection port. Use clamps when performing tubing and injection cap changes. If a CVC access must be open to air, instruct the patient to perform the Valsalva maneuver, if medically possible. Discontinue all lines carefully (see Chapter 4).

Treatment: Treatment for air emboli must be immediate. The patient is placed on his or her left side, with the head lower than the heart (Trendelenburg position); this position allows air to rise into the right atrium and away from the pulmonic valve. If the air is already in the right ventricle, repositioning moves the air to the lower apex of the right ventricle, allowing blood to flow again. Oxygen is usually administered. Identify and correct the cause of air entry as quickly as possible. Do not leave the patient until all symptoms are resolved.

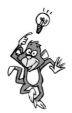

Do You UNDERSTAND?

DIRECTIONS: **Match the causes of air emboli in Column A with the methods of prevention in Column B.**

Column A

1. _____ CVC disconnected tubing
2. _____ Bolus of air through new tubing
3. _____ Air enters vessel through CVC removal track
4. _____ Changing a cap on a catheter, the patient taking a deep breath
5. _____ A hole developing in the external portion

Column B

a. Instruct the patient in the Valsalva maneuver for open systems.
b. Use clamps when necessary.
c. Always prime new tubing.
d. Use Leur connectors or tape all junctions.
e. Use antimicrobial ointment on discontinuation of a nontunneled CVC or CVCs, PICCs, and midlines, along with occlusive pressure dressing.

What IS an Allergic Reaction and Mast Cell Activation Syndrome?

An allergy is a systemic response in which the body reacts with unusual sensitivity to a foreign body or substance. Allergic responses to foreign materials can be reflected in complications such as mast cell activation syndrome,

Answers: 1. d; 2. c; 3. e; 4. a; 5. b.

anaphylactic reactions, or catheter material reactions, or they can be as simple as local site irritation.

What You NEED TO KNOW

Allergic responses are caused by hypersensitivity of the immune system in response to foreign material or other substances. Allergic vasculitis is a condition that occurs from inflammation and damage to blood vessels from an allergic response to a foreign agent or drug. The reaction time of an allergy can vary, as can the area affected. Although most allergic reactions occur within seconds or minutes of contact with a sensitized agent, some can occur after days or weeks.

Mast cell activation syndrome is caused by the activation of the body's immune response to a foreign material. Just under the skin are capillaries that carry blood with circulating red and white blood cells. The tissues of the dermis house specialized immune cells, referred to as mast cells. Any type of allergic reaction is the result of the response of mast cells to an allergen. When a foreign material is inserted into the body, rejection can occur from the activation of the mast cells. The end result of mast cell activation is a local inflammatory response (e.g., redness, tissue swelling) and can lead to itching, tearing eyes, welt formation, wheezing, bronchospasm, vasovagal-type responses, and fainting.

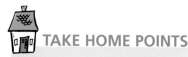

TAKE HOME POINTS

Vasovagal response includes vagus nerve parasympathetic response on blood vessels. This response includes involuntary actions on the heart, lungs, and digestive tract.

What You DO

Prevention: Prevention of the syndrome may not be possible. Careful history documentation can help others to be alert to the potential for this problem.

Treatment: Treatment for mast cell activation is determined by the intensity of the allergic response. Antihistamines will usually manage the inflammation caused by the mast cell degranulation. In severe situations, maintain the airway; the physician may order adrenaline or epinephrine. Mast cell activation syndrome may appear as a catheter material reaction or vasovagal responses.

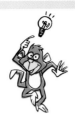

Do You UNDERSTAND?

DIRECTIONS: Each block has letters that are part of a word.
Unscramble the BLOCKS and rearrange letters to form
words to reveal the message.

EAT	T FO	TR	IS DE	MEN	LLE	RG	R MA
ST CE	TIVA	TION	TER	ITY	ED B	Y TH	ESP
ONSE	OF	ENS	THE A	E INT	LL AC	IC R	MIN

1. Treatment __ __ __   __ __ __ __ cell __ __ __ __ __ __ __ __ __ __ __

__ __ __ __ __ __ __ __ __ __ __ __ __ __ __ __ __ intensity

__ __ the __ __ __ __ __ __ __ __ __ __ __ __ __ __ __ __.

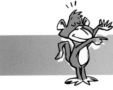

What IS Circulatory Overload and Pulmonary Edema?

Circulatory overload refers to an excessive fluid volume in the bloodstream,
which can lead to pulmonary edema. Pulmonary edema is the accumulation
of fluid in the lung.

What You NEED TO KNOW

Rapid infusion of large volumes of fluid rapidly increases the circulating blood volume, which increases venous pressure. Then the left ventricle cannot move added blood into veins, leading to venous stasis, which will cause peripheral edema. Eventually, fluid will back up into the lungs. Then the capillary walls of the lungs will leak fluid, and this fluid will then fill alveoli.

Circulatory overload can also occur with the following:

- Infusing excessive amounts of sodium chloride solutions
- Large volume infusions running over multiple days
- Rapid fluid infusion into patients with compromised cardiac, liver, or renal status

Symptoms of circulatory overload and impending pulmonary edema include rapid weight gain, edema, engorged peripheral veins, neck vein distention, increased blood pressure, wide variance between intake and output, crackles in lung fields, and shortness of breath. Patient's typically become anxious as symptoms develop.

> **Never play "catch-up" when an infusion falls behind. Monitor the patient's weight and report any rapid weight gain greater than 2 pounds.**

What You DO

Prevention: Preventive measures include using flow-controlled IV administration sets or infusion pumps, using the correct tubing in a pump, closing all clamps before removing pump tubing from the pump, frequent assessment of the infusion rate settings, and appropriate patient monitoring. Any weight gain in the patient should be reported.

- 2% weight gain: mild fluid volume excess
- 5% weight gain: moderate fluid volume excess
- 8% weight gain: severe fluid volume excess

Assessment: Assess neck veins for distention from the top of the sternum to the angle of the jaw. Know the patient's cardiovascular and renal history. Monitor intake and output.

Treatment: Treatment of circulatory overload is to place the patient in an upright position with feet dependent (semi-Fowler's position), administer oxygen and diuretics as prescribed, and reduce fluid intake. Monitor the patient for positive response to treatment and document results.

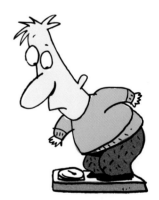

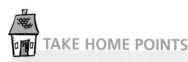
TAKE HOME POINTS

Rapid gain of 2.2 pounds is equal to 1 liter of fluid. Peripheral edema is not usually obvious until 5 to 10 pounds of fluid is retained.

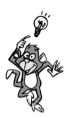

Do You UNDERSTAND?

DIRECTIONS: **Find and circle the following words (with no space between words).**

accumulation	distention	fluid restrict	overload
anxious	diuretic	infusion	oxygen
cardiac	edema	intake	pulmonary
circulatory	engorged veins	lung	sob
compromise	excessive	monitoring	swelling
crackles	fluid	output	weight gain

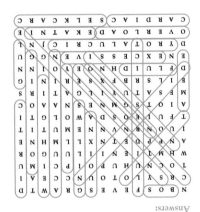

Answers:

```
N  B  O  S  F  E  V  E  S  G  R  A  W  T  D
C  R  S  Y  L  O  T  O  U  N  C  C  E  A  I
T  O  C  N  U  H  U  P  O  I  P  C  I  M  U
W  H  M  T  I  E  N  I  I  L  U  U  G  O  R
A  N  P  P  D  E  T  N  X  L  L  M  H  N  E
I  U  O  N  R  N  V  N  N  E  M  U  T  I  T
T  F  U  I  E  O  S  D  A  W  O  L  G  T  I
A  I  O  T  S  G  M  N  E  S  N  A  A  O  C
M  F  S  A  T  U  Y  I  L  G  A  T  I  R  S
E  I  L  S  R  B  F  X  S  E  R  I  N  I  G
D  F  L  U  I  D  H  N  O  E  Y  O  I  N  N
E  N  E  X  C  E  S  S  I  V  E  N  G  G  U
D  Y  R  O  T  A  L  U  C  R  I  C  J  N  L
O  V  E  R  L  O  A  D  E  K  A  T  N  I  E
C  A  R  D  I  A  C  S  E  L  K  C  A  R  C
```

DIRECTIONS: The letters of the message can be found between the words found in the puzzle on page 148. Once the word search is solved and all the words are found, the hidden message will be revealed.

__ __ __ __ __   __ __ __ __   __ __   __ __ __ __ __

__ __   __ __ __ __   __ __   __ __ __ __ __ __ __ __

__ __ __ __ __   __ __ __ __ __ __ __.

What IS Pneumothorax?

Pneumothorax is when air enters the pleural space and causes the lung to collapse. Pneumothorax can occur during insertion of a CVC.

What You NEED TO KNOW

The lung is punctured, which allows air to enter the pleural space, causing the lung to collapse. The puncture is usually small, and the lung usually collapses only partially. Complication symptoms are generally not seen until after the procedure has been completed. The patient may be asymptomatic for some time, with a gradual onset of symptoms. These symptoms include:

- Chest pain
- Shortness of breath
- Cyanosis
- Decreased or absent breath sounds on side of CVC
- Confusion
- Tachycardia
- Painful inspiration

Answer: **Never try to catch up when an infusion falls behind.**

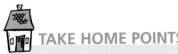

TAKE HOME POINTS

Sudden shortness of breath occurring in conjunction with a CVC insertion may denote a puncture of a lobe of the lung (i.e., pneumothorax).

What You DO

Prevention: Prevention includes proper patient teaching before CVC insertion. For patients who are unable to cooperate or are extremely anxious, the nurse may need to discuss the use of a sedative with the physician before insertion. It is also very important to have the patient in the proper position when the catheter is being inserted.

Treatment: When symptoms occur (may be during or after the insertion process), notify the physician. The patient will be anxious. Place the patient in the Fowler's position. Administer oxygen as prescribed. An x-ray of the chest will be done to confirm the diagnosis. A chest tube may be needed to reinflate the lung.

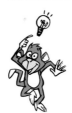

Do You UNDERSTAND?

DIRECTIONS: Unscramble each of the clue words to reveal the symptoms of pneumothorax. Take the letters that appear in the circles and unscramble them for the final message.

HYICATDARCA

HETCS NAPI

SOYCAINS

NOFCOSNUI

RESSOTNSH FO TAHREB

ETANIYX

PAINLFU PSNOINIARIT

SBTANE BATREH SDNOSU

[grid boxes with W and V]

[grid boxes with M and D]

[grid boxes with M]

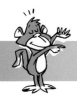

What IS Hemorrhage Associated with Central Venous Devices?

Hemorrhage is excessive bleeding. Hemorrhage from an access device can occur on insertion or removal or from accidental disconnection of the device.

What You NEED TO KNOW

Hemorrhage from a CVC is rare. Causes of hemorrhage from an insertion site include traumatic insertion, use of a large-gauge introducer, or lack of an adequate pressure dressing. Awareness of anticoagulant medication use and laboratory baseline values for the patient can assist in heightening the awareness of a patient's potential for hemorrhage. Episodes of excessive blood loss (exsanguinations) from a patient have resulted from loose tubing connections, accidental disconnection, or failure to apply a clamp to the CVC.

TAKE HOME POINTS

Medications that have anticoagulant properties include aspirin, Coumadin, NSAIDs, heparin, vitamin E, and warfarin.

What You DO

Prevention: Use pressure dressings. Limiting patient activity for the first 24 hours after insertion or removal helps minimize bleeding at the site. Instruct the patient that activity limitations will enable the insertion site to heal. Heavy pressure dressings are indicated for insertions with gauge sizes greater than 16 gauge. To prevent accidental blood loss through the catheter, always close clamps when the CVC is not in use. Use only Leur lock connections with CVCs. Always assess connections to ensure that they are secure.

Treatment: Treatment of hemorrhage includes reinforcing of the dressing, elevating the insertion site (if applicable), manual pressure to the insertion site, and, possibly, using coagulating foams. Excessive bleeding that does not resolve should be reported to the physician. Excessive bruising or pain can be a sign of venous perforation and should be reported to the physician immediately.

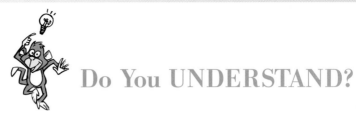

Do You UNDERSTAND?

DIRECTIONS: Solve a phrase by placing the correct letters in the boxes. Each letter appears in the same column but above or below where it should be. The solver must put the letters back in the grid and rebuild the phrase. HINT: When does hemorrhage occur most often?

	H		O						
					O				
O		O							
					O		O		
	R								

```
S  E  O     V  A  A
L  M  R  R  I  C  L     R
N  R  A  M  W  I  O  C     C
I  H  E  E  N  O  O  H  N  U  O  R
F  O  C  L  O  T  R  N  G  G  E  V  C
```

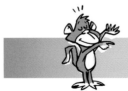

What IS an Occlusion?

Any time a CVC will not flush or allow flow, the device is considered occluded. Occlusions are caused by mechanical, drug, or blood obstructions. CVC occlusions are a common problem, especially with small-gauge catheters, such as PICC lines.

What You NEED TO KNOW

Mechanical Occlusions

Mechanical occlusions are caused by improper function of some part of the administration setup, the dressing, or the catheter that prevents flow. Some occlusions are simple to identify, such as kinks and closed clamps (see Chapter 3), but others are less obvious and are caused internally through positioning of the catheter.

Drug-Precipitate Occlusions

Physical incompatibilities occur when one drug is mixed with other drugs or solutions to produce a precipitate. This condition is seen as a visible precipitate, haze, or cloudiness. The crystals, seen as flakes or floating solids separated from the solution, can completely occlude a CVC. Drug precipitates usually occur because they are administered concurrently or in close succession without proper flushing between them through the same IV line.

Drugs Physically Incompatible with Heparin

- alteplase (Activase)
- amikacin (Amikin)
- amiodarone (Cordarone)
- ampicillin sodium
- atropine
- cephalothin sodium (Keflin)
- chlorpromazine (Thorazine)
- ciprofloxacin (Cipro)
- dacarbazine (DTIC)
- daunorubicin HCL
- diazepam (valium)
- diltiazem (Cardizem)
- dobutamine (Dobutrex)
- doxorubicin (Adriamycin)
- doxycycline (Vibramycin)
- droperidol (Inapsine)
- erythromycin
- filgrastim (Neupogen)
- gentamicin
- haloperidol (Haldol)
- idarubicin (Idamycin)
- kanamycin (Kantrex)
- levorphanol
- meperidine HCL (Demerol)
- methotrimeprazine (Levoprome)
- mitoxantrone HCL (Novantrone)
- netilmicin (Netromycin)
- phenytoin (Dilantin)
- promazine HCL
- promethazine (Phenergan)
- quinidine gluconate
- streptomycin sulfate
- teniposide (VM-26)
- tobramycin (Nebcin, Tobrex)
- triflupromazine (Vesprin)
- vancomycin

TAKE HOME POINTS

Flush CVCs with 5% Dextrose in water (D₅W) when giving alkaline drugs such as amphotericin B and Dilantin IV.

The solubility of a drug may be determined by the pH. Some drugs require an acidic or alkaline environment to remain in solution. When this environment is abruptly altered by a medication or solution, a precipitate can be formed. Alkaline drugs such as amphotericin, phenytoin (Dilantin), ampicillin, and ganciclovir result in precipitates when mixed with low-pH solutions, as with saline, vancomycin, morphine, doxycycline, and promethazine (Phenergan). In TPN, calcium and phosphates can form insoluble salts that form a precipitate.

Administration of lipids causes buildup of fats, over time, within the CVC. When lipids come in contact with blood, a substance referred to as sludge is formed, which can occlude the catheter.

Blood Occlusions

Fibrin can build up inside the catheter (intraluminal) as a result of:

- Improper or inconsistent flushing
- Increased venous pressure found with excessive coughing, vomiting, or crying
- Pump malfunction
- Blood reflux
- Extremely low keep vein open (KVO) rates with ambulatory pumps

A blood occlusion occurs when a clot completely occludes the lumen of the catheter. Blood occlusions can occur suddenly, as when the IV solution runs dry and the blood backs up into the tubing, or over time, as blood residue builds up in the catheter lumen, causing sluggish flow. Failure to correctly flush is a common cause of blood occlusions. (See Chapter 4 on flushing.)

Signs of occlusion are related to buildup of materials within the CVC or external pressure on the catheter. These signs include:

- Decreased or sluggish infusion rate
- Increased resistance when flushing
- Leaking from the insertion site
- Inability to withdraw blood

TAKE HOME POINTS

The primary causes for drug or blood occlusions include:
- Inappropriate flushing solutions
- Inadequate flushing
- Omission or poor scheduling of flushing

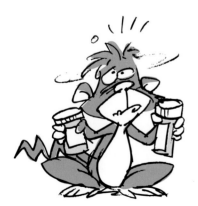

What You DO

Prevention: The vast majority of occlusions of CVCs can be prevented. Flushing is vital to prevent occlusion. Use saline–administer medication–saline (SAS) method or saline–administer medication–saline–heparinized saline

(SASH) method of flushing when administering medications (see Chapter 2). The amount of flush will vary from one institution to the next; follow the flushing policy of the facility. Unlike peripheral catheters, heparinized saline is commonly instilled into open-ended catheters. The manufacturers of valved catheters and some positive-pressure end caps state that their products do not require the final heparinized saline flush.

Knowledge of drug-solution interactions is critical to prevent precipitates. Speak with a pharmacist with any drug interaction questions. Inspect all solutions before infusion. Assess for precipitates, discoloration, and leaks in the bag. Precipitates will be visible, floating in the IV bags. Any discoloration, leaks, or particulate matter in an IV solution require pharmacy contact and probable disposal of the solution. Valve catheters or pressure-valve end caps (e.g., Catheter Innovations PasV™ products, Bard Access System's Groshong® catheter, Abbott/ICU Medical's CLC 2000 pressure-end caps) are designed to reduce blood entry into the catheter. Proper flushing, including schedule, amount, and push-pause technique, is the best way to prevent drug contact. Flushing is performed daily, even on continuous infusions, to help reduce buildup of materials within a CVC. Teach other staff members the steps of prevention with CVCs, thus ensuring continuity of care and improved outcomes for patients.

Assessment: Determining the type of occlusion is the first step to correcting the problem successfully. If the wrong declotting agent is used, it will not work. First investigate when the device was last functioning, who discovered the problem, and what they were doing with the CVC. This knowledge will uncover whether the occlusion is mechanical, drug related, or a clotted line. If the clot is fibrin, a thrombolytic agent is used. However, if the obstruction is caused by a drug precipitate or sludge, the thrombolytic will not work.

Knowledge about drug-solution interactions is important if precipitates are to be prevented. If questions about drug interaction arise, communication with a pharmacist is necessary. Because new drugs are constantly coming into use, pharmacists are the best resource for up-to-date information. Proper flushing (including schedule, amount, and technique) is the best way to prevent the contact between drugs.

Treatment: Resolution of occlusions may be as simple as changing the tubing and choosing the appropriate flushing procedure or as invasive as replacing the CVC. Mechanical occlusions can usually be resolved with identification of the problem. When a drug precipitate is suspected, the solution environment must be returned to the pH required by the original drug. Hydrochloric acid returns the solution to an acidic environment, and sodium bicarbonate returns the solution to an alkaline environment. If sludge is

TAKE HOME POINTS

Use the SASH or SAS method of flushing when administering medications.
Saline–**A**dminister medication–
Saline–**H**eparinized saline.
OR
Saline–**A**dminister medication–**S**aline

TAKE HOME POINTS

Do not assume an occluded catheter is occluded with blood.

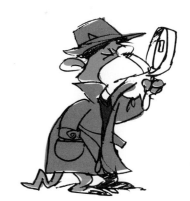

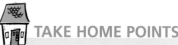

TAKE HOME POINTS

Thrombolytics are more expensive than are drug precipitate–clearing solutions.

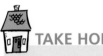

suspected, then ethyl alcohol (ETOH) is the clearing agent. Ask the institution's pharmacist for assistance in obtaining the appropriate declotting agent when attempting to dissolve drug or sludge precipitates. When blood is the cause, a thrombolytic such as alteplase (Cath-Flo) is used.

Declotting agents are instilled into the catheter using the institution procedure, left in place for the prescribed period, and then aspirated. If fibrin is suggested, it is important to initiate the declotting procedure at the earliest opportunity, because the older the clot, the more resistant to treatment it becomes. In addition, clots are known to be a haven for bacteria, which can lead to catheter infection.

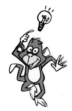

Do You UNDERSTAND?

DIRECTIONS: Complete the crossword puzzle on the following page.

Across

2. A syndrome that occurs with the pressure from the first rib on the clavicle compressing a catheter, resulting in intermittent occlusion
3. Alteplase
7. A mechanism added to a catheter designed to reduce blood backup in the catheter and reduce the need for heparin
8. An interaction of chemicals in solution that results in flakes, crystals, or snowlike particles
9. The acid or basic value of the solution or drug
11. Slower rate of infusion than was originally established; may be intermittent flow

Down

1. Type of obstruction of the catheter, suture, or tubing
3. A current, or swirling of solution, created with push-pause-push action in conjunction with a catheter, syringe, and flushing
4. Blocked off
5. Not mixing, such as oil and water
6. A method to clear and clean out a catheter after infusions, using isotonic solutions such as sterile normal saline or dextrose in water
10. Protein derived from fibrinogen in the presence of thrombin, which forms a coating or strands as part of the blood clot
12. A fat solution

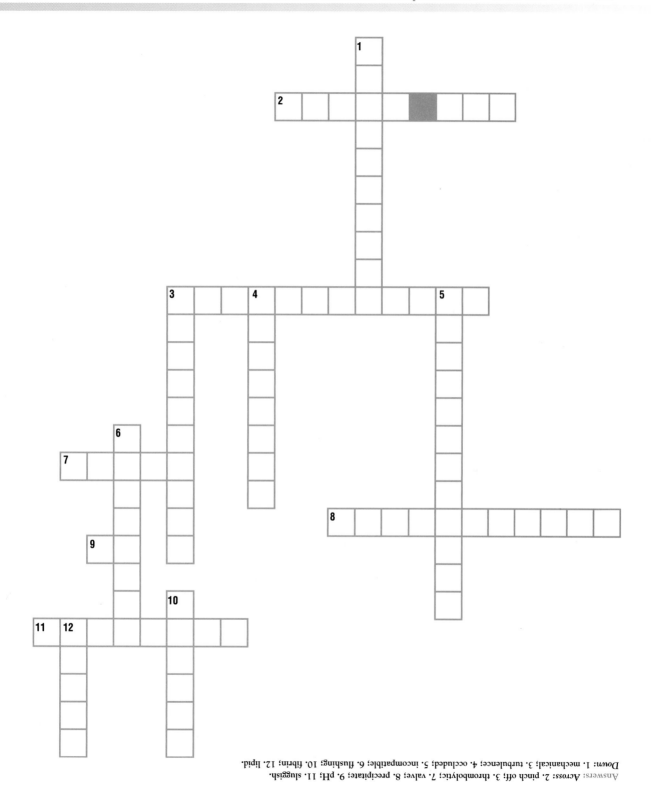

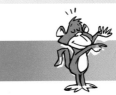

What IS Catheter Damage?

CVCs are made of silicone or polyurethane, each breakable if given adequate tension or force on the line. Most damage occurs externally when the external portion is pulled too hard, compressed over and over, stretched to the point of breaking, or cut. Internal breakage can occur with pinch-off syndrome, forceful flushing, or a manufacturer defect in the CVC.

What You NEED TO KNOW

⚠ External chest braces can constantly hit implanted ports during body movement, causing the port to break apart, which can lead to catheter embolism.

Causes of catheter breakage are stretching (e.g., a patient goes to the bathroom and forgets the IV pump; the catheter and tubing stretch, breaking or pulling out somewhere between the bed and bathroom), excess torsion that results in cracking, forceful flushing, high-pressure injectors, breakage during discontinuation of a catheter, improper handling of the catheter during dressing changes, accidental cutting of the catheter while using scissors, or using a clamp not suited for the catheter. Repeated flexing of the hub-catheter connection can weaken the joint, and it can eventually break. External damage is more common with catheters made out of silicone. Polyurethane catheters may crack with repetitive motion. Cracking of catheters results in splits and breaks that may completely separate the catheter.

Internal damage can occur with the pinch-off syndrome (i.e., repetitive compression with normal shoulder and arm movement that can result in catheter fracture) and increased pressure associated with flushing that resulted from some type of occlusion (see color plate 17).

By far, the most common cause of catheter damage is exerting too much force on a syringe plunger while flushing a catheter that is partially occluded. The damage can be a small rupture as in a hole, or the entire catheter can break off and become a catheter embolism. Pressure injectors, used in radiologic procedures that require continuous visualization with contrast, can easily create enough pressure to rupture a CVC. Smaller CVCs, such as PICCs, Broviac® catheters, and softer silicone CVCs (e.g., Hickman®), have lower burst pressures and are more susceptible to rupture than polyurethane catheters (e.g., Groshong®). Assess the CVC manufacturer's package insert for the burst pressure on specific devices. Any pressure injector exceeding the levels recommended by the manufacturer of a CVC may cause breakage of the device.

Fracture can occur when removing a catheter. Venospasm or the presence of a thrombus along the catheter can impede removal of a catheter. Fibrin buildup on the surface of the catheter may fold with a clump, resulting in increased difficulty to remove the catheter (see color plate 18).

Another cause of catheter shearing or fracture can occur during insertion. Through-the-needle insertion technique carries the risk of catheter shearing if the catheter is pulled back through the needle during the insertion procedure (catheter may catch on the needle bevel and be cut). The risk is especially high when the catheter is silicone.

Signs of catheter fracture include:

- The presence of a hub without a catheter
- Patient reports a popping sensation after flushing
- Part of the catheter falls on the floor
- Unusual points of swelling along upper arm venous pathway (PICC)
- Swelling under the skin
- Signs of infiltration with a CVC
- Leaking at the insertion site without thrombosis
- Saturated dressing
- Leaking during flushing
- Inadequate catheter length discovered after the catheter has been removed
- Chest pain (may indicate break of implanted port catheters); may have sudden onset
- Shortness of breath
- Chest wall swelling or feeling of fullness with infusion at port pocket or vein insertion site
- Pain in shoulder not associated with swelling
- Cardiac arrhythmias, usually ventricular
- Extra heart sound
- Palpitation
- Cough
- Paresthesia of arm on side of catheter
- X-ray confirming catheter fragment

TAKE HOME POINTS

Pressure injectors are best used with short peripheral IV devices.

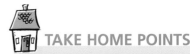

TAKE HOME POINTS

The greater the resistance felt with flushing, the greater the risk of rupture. Avoid flushing against resistance with any size syringe (see Chapter 4).

Catheter Fracture

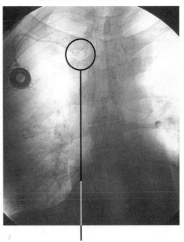

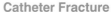

Fracture

What You DO

Prevention: Prevention focuses on safe flushing practices, adequate dressing management, catheter securement (see Chapter 4), and patient-staff education. Radiology departments must ensure that high-pressure injectors are not used on CVCs unless within the manufacturer's specifications for safe pressure with the device. When removing PICCs, do not apply excessive tension (see Chapter 4).

Assessment: If catheter damage occurs, it is important to determine the cause of the damage. This knowledge will help prevent the problem from occurring again. Identify pinch-off syndrome early; intermittent occlusion is not a normal function. At the first sign of resistance during flushing or catheter removal, stop and evaluate the situation. If the problem cannot be resolved (see Chapter 4), notify the physician of the problem and then proceed with additional measures designed to repair or remove the catheter. Symptoms of catheter damage, fracture, or shearing must be reported to the physician immediately. If internal damage is suspected, dye studies in x-ray will be the best diagnostic tool. Catheter fragments lost in the central circulation may go to the right atrium, ventricles, or commonly, the pulmonary artery, making retrieval difficult. Retrieval of fragments is possible only through radiologic and surgical intervention.

Treatment: Actions recommended for sudden breakage of a catheter that is threaded up the arm and into the central circulation (PICC line), include the application of a tourniquet on the upper arm near the shoulder. The rationale of tourniquet application is to hold the catheter fragment in the periphery long enough for easy retrieval.

TAKE HOME POINTS

Less than one third of patients exhibit signs and symptoms of catheter fracture. This lack of evidence is because of the presence of few sensory nerve endings in the vascular endothelium and endocardium where the catheter segment migrates.

TAKE HOME POINTS

- Always apply minimal force to the syringe to activate a flush. Do not yield to the natural tendency to apply more pressure with the thumb when resistance is felt.
- Catheter breakage can be prevented in many cases through education of patients and staff.
- Safe flushing practices with larger syringes, adequate catheter securement, and careful removal of catheters can significantly reduce the incidence of catheter breakage with CVCs.

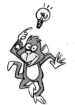

Do You UNDERSTAND?

DIRECTIONS: Choose a letter to complete a word. Find the number below the chosen letter (newly filled-in blank). Write the number in the block under the printed letter in the decoding line for reference. Then fill in all the numbered blanks that match with the letter. Repeat the process until the phrase is complete.

A	B	C	D	E	F	G	H	I	J	K	L	M	N	O	P	Q	R	S	T	U	V	W	X	Y	Z
			24				12										18	23							

```
 T     E        R  E     T  E  R     T     E
23  5  24     10 18 24  8 23 24 18   23  5 24

 R  E     I     T              E        E     T        I  T
18 24  7 12  7 23  8    16  4 24    11 24  3 23    15 12 23  5

                   I           T     E        R  E     T  E  R
11  3 14  7  5 12 16 10      23  5 24       10 18 24  8 23 24 18

 T     E     R  I                    R        T     R  E
23  5 24    18 12  7 25    21 11    18 14 22 23 14 18 24
```

What IS Catheter Malpositioning and Migration?

Central venous devices are inserted with the terminal tip in the SVC or inferior vena cava (IVC). When insertion misses the desired SVC or IVC, or when patient activities cause excess tip movement into the jugular vein, the catheter is considered malpositioned.

What You NEED TO KNOW

The position of all CVCs is confirmed by x-ray before infusion of medications or solutions. Catheter migration can be internal or external. Internal catheter migration occurs when a catheter moves from the confirmed terminal tip–placement location (e.g., into the right atrium, up the jugular vein, across into the opposite subclavian vein). External catheter migration is when a catheter comes out externally and is no longer in the confirmed terminal tip–placement location. Catheters can malposition at any time. Patients with coughing, vomiting, and other causes of increased inner thoracic pressure can cause the CVC to malposition in the jugular vein or subclavian vein. Malpositioned CVCs in jugular-placed lines do not always have symptoms.

Symptoms of a malpositioned catheter in the jugular vein include:
- Buzzing in the ear
- Rushing water sounds
- Tingling or funny feeling in the neck
- Inability to withdraw blood from the catheter
- A gurgling sound heard by the patient during the flush procedure
- Headache, pain, swelling in neck or shoulder area

Catheter migration may have symptoms of phlebitis, thrombosis, jugular symptoms, coughing, feeling of fullness, chest pain, vague back pain, shoulder pain, or arrhythmias (if being monitored), or there may be no symptoms at all.

What You DO

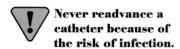

Never readvance a catheter because of the risk of infection.

Radiologic examination of a CVC is necessary if catheter malpositioning or migration is suspected. Prevention involves adequate securement to maintain proper positioning, measurement of external catheter length with each dressing change, and patient education on signs and symptoms of malpositioning or migration. Once a line has migrated out of the insertion site, secure the catheter.

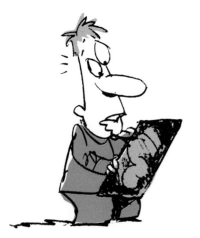

Catheter Migration

Catheter tip —

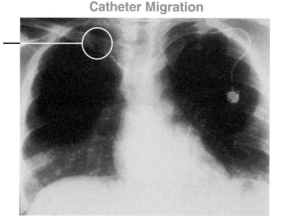

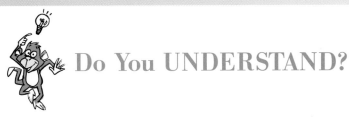

Do You UNDERSTAND?

DIRECTIONS: Choose a letter to complete a word. Find the number
below the chosen letter (newly filled-in blank). Write
the number in the block under the printed letter in the
decoding line for reference. Then fill in all the numbered blanks that match with the letter. Repeat the
process until the phrase is complete.

A	B	C	D	E	F	G	H	I	J	K	L	M	N	O	P	Q	R	S	T	U	V	W	X	Y	Z
8		23		11			18	24			26	19	10				6		20						

```
I   N  T  E  R  N  A  L     C  A  T  H  E  T  E  R
24  10 20 11 6  10 8  26    23 8  20 18 11 20 11 6
M   I  _  R  A  T  I  _  N     _  C  C  _  R  _     _  H  E  N
19  24 12 6  8  20 24 16 10    16 23 23 17 6  4     15 18 11 10
T   H  E     C  A  T  H  E  T  E  R     T  I  _
20  18 11    23 8  20 18 11 20 11 6     20 24 1
M   _  E  _  _  R  _  M     T  H  E
19  16 5  11 4     14 6  16 19    20 18 11
C   N  _  I  R  M  E  _     T  E  R  M  I  N  A  L
23  16 10 14 24 6  19 11 2     20 11 6  19 24 10 8  26
T   I  _  L  _  C  A  T  I  _  N.  E  _  T  E  R  N  A  L
20  24 1  26 16 23 8  20 24 16 10  11 21 20 11 6  10 8  26
C   A  T  H  E  T  E  R     M  I  _  R  A  T  I  _  N
23  8  20 18 11 20 11 6     19 24 12 6  8  20 24 16 10
I   _  _  H  E  N     A     C  A  T  H  E  T  E  R
24  4     15 18 11 10    8     23 8  20 18 11 20 11 6
C   _  M  E  _  _  _  T     E  _  T  E  R  N  A  L  L  _
23  16 19 11 4     16 17 20    11 21 20 11 6  10 8  26 26 25
A   N  _  I  _  N     L  _  N     E  R  _  I  N
8   10 2  24 4     10 16    26 16 10 12    11 6     24 10
T   H  E     C  _  N  _  I  R  M  E  _
20  18 11    23 16 10 14 24 6  19 11 2
L   _  C  A  T  I  _  N     _  R  _  T  I  _
26  16 23 8  20 24 16 10    14 16 6     20 24 1
      _  I  T  I  _  N.  C  A  T  H  E  T  E  R  _
1    16 4  24 20 24 16 10  23 8  20 18 11 20 11 6  4
C   A  N  _  M  A  L  _  _  I  T  I  _  N     A  T
23  8  10 19 8  26 1  16 4  24 20 24 16 10    8  20
A   N  _     T  I  M  E.
8   10 25    20 24 19 11
```

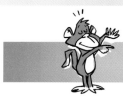

What IS Pinch-Off Syndrome?

Pinch-off syndrome is the compression of a central catheter inserted into the subclavian vein by the clavicle and first rib. The incident rate is 0.1% to 5.0% of subclavian-placed catheters. Between 20% and 40% of these catheters will shear and migrate. Approximately 80% of all catheters that separate are a result of pinch-off syndrome. Catheter fracture can occur with any catheter, but it is more prevalent with tunneled and implanted catheters.

What You NEED TO KNOW

Improper placement is the primary cause of pinch-off syndrome. Placing the catheter medially to the midclavicular line positions the catheter in the clavicle space. Respirations and the weight of the shoulder cause repeated compression of the catheter between the clavicle and the first rib.

The distance between the first rib and clavicle is narrower in women than in men. This difference increases the potential for pinch-off syndrome in small women.

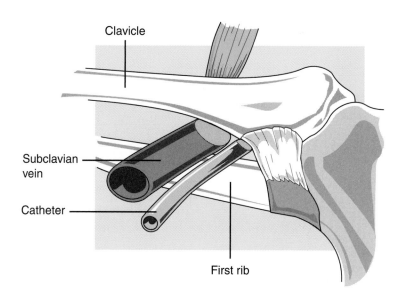

Clavicle

Subclavian vein

Catheter

First rib

The ideal location for subclavian insertion is at, or lateral to, the midclavicular line.

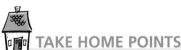

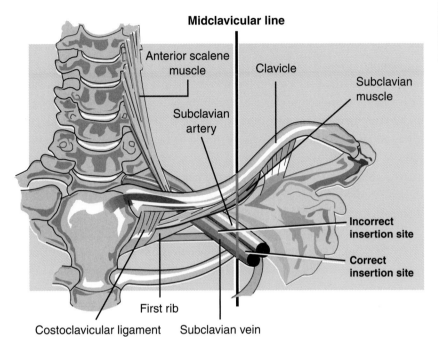

Midclavicular line

Anterior scalene muscle

Clavicle

Subclavian artery

Subclavian muscle

Incorrect insertion site

Correct insertion site

First rib

Costoclavicular ligament   Subclavian vein

Signs and symptoms of pinch-off syndrome are:
- Difficulty with blood aspiration or loss of blood return
- Positional catheter with blood draws that is corrected by turning of the head or lifting the arm up
- "Ballooning out" of the catheter when flushed
- Resistance to flushing that improves with turning the head or lifting the arm
- Occlusion relieved by rolling the shoulder or raising the arm on the same side as the catheter
- Withdrawal occlusion that is sudden, intermittent, or both (may be confused with catheter occlusion caused by thrombin)
- Alarm sounding on an electronic infusion device

Symptoms of pinch-off syndrome are seen on average at 5 days with continuous infusions and 120 days with intermittent infusions.

When the catheter is improperly positioned, repeated mechanical friction and compression can lead to catheter fracture. Participation in sports such as golf, basketball, weight lifting, and hiking with backpacks can increase catheter exposure to repeated compression.

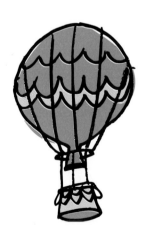

Relieved Pinch-Off

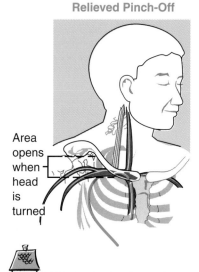

Area opens when head is turned

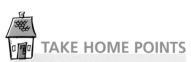

TAKE HOME POINTS

Occlusions that are a result of fibrin or drug precipitates will not resolve with position change.

TAKE HOME POINTS

Investigate all changes in catheter function.

What You DO

Prevention: Although the best way to prevent pinch-off syndrome involves the manner in which the CVC is inserted, some preventative actions can be taken. One method is to avoid positioning the patient before insertion in such a way as to widen the clavicle–first rib angle (e.g., placing a rolled towel under the shoulder on the insertion side). A blood return should be achieved after insertion. The patient should be taught the signs and symptoms of pinch-off syndrome, and the physician's instructions on sporting activities should be reinforced. When the nurse experiences any changes in catheter performance, he or she should investigate the cause. Pinch-off syndrome may suggest the need for change in catheter function.

Assessment: When intermittent infusion or blood withdrawal occurs, pinch off should be considered. Since catheter occlusion can have different causes, it is important to do a thorough assessment to determine the cause of the problem. Pinch off is relieved by changing the patient's position in such a way as to widen the first rib and clavicle area (i.e., raising the arm, laying down or turning the head away from the catheter insertion site).

When the catheter is lying against the vein wall (i.e., when the patient has been sleeping, coughing, or performing a Valsalva maneuver), when medically appropriate, or when the patient is sitting upright, the catheter will usually move away from the wall, alleviating the problem. Any signs or symptoms that are identified must be documented so that assessment of changes can be made over time. Signs and symptoms should be communicated to the physician.

Treatment: A chest x-ray is required to confirm pinch-off syndrome. The patient's arms must remain at the side during the x-ray procedure. Raising the arms and rolling them forward are routine with chest x-rays, which will correct the compression and make the diagnosis impossible. Fluoroscopy with contrast dye can determine catheter integrity. The patient should sit upright with arms down by the sides. Any distortion observed on either of these examinations should be evaluated. Catheters identified with pinch-off syndrome should be removed as soon as possible, which will prevent catheter fracture.

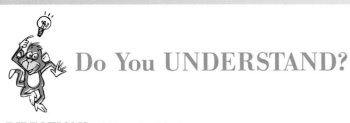

Do You UNDERSTAND?

DIRECTIONS: **Fill in the blanks.**

1. _____   _____ should be considered when catheter malfunction is relieved by asking the patient to raise his or her hands above the head.

2. _____   _____ can result if pinch-off syndrome is not identified early.

3. _____   _____ is the primary cause of pinch-off syndrome.

DIRECTIONS: **Identify the following statements as *true* (T) or *false* (F).**

4. _____ It is best to position the patient to widen the angle between the first rib and clavicle for subclavian catheter insertion.

5. _____ Activities such as golf and backpacking can increase the risk for pinch-off syndrome in a patient with an implanted port.

DIRECTIONS: **Select the best answer.**

6. _____ The nurse has been able to draw blood easily for several days, and then he or she is unable to do so unless the patient turns his or her head. What should the nurse do?

   a. Change the plan of care to include changing head position to obtain blood return.

   b. Notify the physician of the problem.

Pediatric Patient

Top Bananas: Chapter 6 Overview

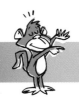

What IS Pediatric IV Therapy?

Inserting and maintaining peripheral intravenous (IV) and central venous catheters (CVCs) is challenging and generates distinctive problems. Pediatric patients are very different from adults in physiology, developmental accomplishments, and ability to cooperate. Successful pediatric IV therapy is founded on an explicit understanding of the child, the caregiver, the environment, and how all these factors affect venipuncture. Additionally, professional IV standards of practice still apply to children, and the nurse should be familiar with these tenets.

What You NEED TO KNOW

Thermoregulation

Children have fewer subcutaneous layers than do adults and can therefore be cold-stressed easily. The vein has only a small amount of connective tissue. Cold children become vasoconstricted. Babies do not shiver; therefore care must be taken to reduce heat loss. Unwrapping a baby can cause heat loss to the surrounding surfaces (convection) and, if placed on a cool surface, the child can lose heat to the surface. Children can lose heat to the air (evaporation). Only the area to be examined should be unwrapped, the surface on which the child is laying should be covered with a nonconductive material (e.g., towel, blanket), the room temperature should be comfortable, and the child should have on one more layer of clothing than the caregiver. The infant uses a thermogenic process involving brown-fat metabolism to provide heat when he or she is cold-stressed. When this process is activated, the baby is prone to acidosis. The nurse must be careful with a febrile child not to provide too much thermal support because this will cause body temperature to continue to rise, and the child may have a febrile seizure.

Pediatric Physiologic, Anatomic, and Developmental Considerations

DEVELOPMENTAL STAGE	AGE	BODY FAT	METABOLISM	SURGERY PREPARATION
Premature infant	< 32 weeks' gestation	No subcutaneous fat	Immature liver and renal function	Infiltration is common because of vein wall fragility and poor catheter stabilization.
Infant	Birth-1 yr	12%	Immature liver and renal function	Do not use parents to restrain infant.
Toddler	1-3 yrs	16%	Immature renal function; mature liver functions	Educate caregiver on process of venipuncture.
Preschool	4-6 yrs	12%	Mature renal and liver function	Prepare for procedure immediately before venipuncture.
School age	6-12 yrs	20%	Mature renal and liver function	Prepare for procedure several hours before venipuncture.
Adolescent	13-19 yrs	20%	Mature renal and liver function	Prepare patient hours-to-days in advance, leaving time for questions.

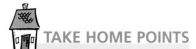

Repeated blood draws can produce hypovolemia.

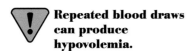

TAKE HOME POINTS

The use of scalp veins may be restricted in some institutions.

Blood Volume

Although the blood volume of a child occupies a larger percentage of the total body weight than that in the adult, the total volume of blood is smaller by comparison. Repeated blood draws can produce hypovolemia. Blood replacement is recommended when a child's blood loss totals 5% to 7% of total blood volume.

Average circulating blood volume is as follows:

- **Premature infant:** 95 ml/kg; example for determining circulating blood volume: 1.5 kg (infant weight) $\times$ 95 = 153 ml of circulating blood volume
- **Term infant:** 80 ml/kg; example for determining circulating blood volume: 3.5 kg (infant weight) $\times$ 80 = 280 ml of circulating blood volume
- **1- to 12-month toddler:** 75 ml/kg
- **1- to 6-year-old preschool child:** 70 ml/kg
- **7-year-old school-age child to 18-year-old adolescent:** 80 ml/kg
- **Adult:** 80 ml/kg; example for determining circulating blood volume: 70 kg $\times$ 80 = 5600 ml of circulating blood volume

Vein Size

The veins of infants and children are much smaller and have less connective tissue compared with those of adults or adolescents. Many conditions and circumstances can make determining vein size difficult, such as cold stress, decreased circulating volume because of dehydration, or the presence of subcutaneous fat in the older infant and some toddlers. **Scalp veins** are used in children up to approximately 18 months of age when hair follicles have matured. Scalp veins are easily visualized and accessed. These veins do not have valves.

Foot veins are used in infants and toddlers up to 2 years of age. These veins are avoided in children who can walk. Foot veins dilate easily, are more easily stabilized for venipuncture, are more visible in chubby infants, and are easy to protect. **Metacarpal veins** of the hands are often the only visible veins of the hand. **Antecubital veins** are used. If the child is chubby, the veins on the forearm may be difficult to identify.

Scalp veins

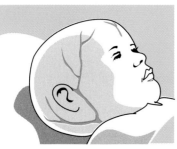

Foot veins

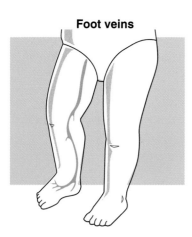

Metacarpal veins

Antecubital veins

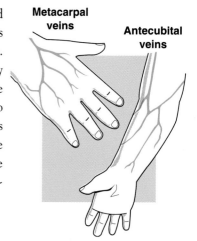

Stress

Any stress, physical or emotional, can adversely affect the venipuncture process in pediatric patients. Any patient, regardless of age, will produce norepinephrine when stressed. To prevent this reaction in the infant or young child, attention must be devoted to providing for the physical and emotional comfort of the child, which means that the nurse must be aware of the interplay of emotions between parent and child, the developmental age of the child, the child's coping methods, and the child's cultural background.

When performing a venipuncture, the goal is to prevent stress in the child that may provide the precursor to adrenaline secretion and generalized vasoconstriction. If the child can relate to the venipuncture activity through play, the process will proceed much smoother.

Helping the child understand why the venipuncture process is necessary and what the child can do to protect the site will empower a child even as young as 2 years of age. It helps if the treatment room is child-friendly—with juvenile printed posters and even child-decorated ceiling tiles and mobiles extending from the ceiling that move with the breezes in the room. Music, whatever type appeals to the child, can help the child relax.

It might help nurses understand the fears of children to imagine that they were 2 to 3 feet tall and that these 5- or 6-foot medical giants were bent on imposing these painful procedures on them—no matter what they say. The IV procedure should be completely explained to the child. Use of age-appropriate education and play are important to help a child understand the necessity for IV therapy.

Ambient Lighting

The lighting in the room should be adjustable, from very bright to totally dark. A bright light, such as an otoscope or a Mag-Light flashlight can be used in darkness to help identify potential veins for venipuncture on small infants and pudgy toddlers. Bright fluorescent lights will also help make veins more obvious on older children.

Air Temperature

Room temperature is a very important part of pediatric venipuncture. If the child is allowed to become chilled, his or her veins will constrict, and the venipuncture process will become extremely difficult.

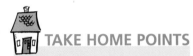

TAKE HOME POINTS

The child's developmental age may not always correspond to the child's chronologic age.

Being too close to strange adults is particularly stressful for children of certain cultures. Hispanic children, for example, are taught not to be directly *en face* with an adult. Some adults can misconstrue this behavior as disrespectful.

TAKE HOME POINTS

- Keep the pediatric patient warm.
- The child's bedroom should provide a safe haven in which hurtful things do not happen.

Privacy

Venipunctures for children should be done in a treatment room. The child's bedroom should be a safe haven. Nothing traumatizing should be done at the bedside. If the treatment room serves more than one function for the nursing unit (e.g., storage area, supply room), the venipuncture should proceed without interruption. If distractions are allowed, the child, the "holder(s)," and the nurse performing the venipuncture can be distracted, even if only for a moment. This momentary distraction can compromise successful venipuncture. Additionally, privacy is not just an adult issue. Every child has the right to privacy during procedures. A telephone is beneficial in the treatment room to summon help when needed, and a "Do Not Disturb" sign is a helpful detail in the treatment room.

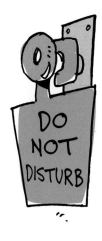

Safety

Venipuncture is a much safer process if the child is placed on one surface and the supplies are placed on a Mayo stand or overbed table. A trash can nearby prevents accumulation of papers and plastic bits that might provide a choking hazard for the child. The room should have clear lanes around the child's surface to prevent injuries to the nurses, holders, and parents. The parent should always have a seat available just in case of potential light-headedness. The parent should also be out of range of any inadvertent kicks from the child.

Presence of Parents

It is in the best interests of the child for the nurse to observe the interaction between parent and child and see how the family relates to each other before the venipuncture process is begun. The parents should be given the option to accompany the child or go to the waiting room as they deem appropriate. The child's emotional comfort is an important component of successful venipuncture. It is not safe to have the parents actively involved in the venipuncture process. The parent can provide enormous support to the child and provide a distraction, but the process itself is the responsibility of the nurse. The child cannot perceive the parent as opposing the venipuncture process. Friction among the nurses and parents is extremely confusing and upsetting to the child. If friction is present between the nurse and the parent, the venipuncture process should be deferred, if possible, to someone more comfortable to the parents. Parental support gets increasingly difficult when people other than parents are the responsible adult in the absence of the parents, such as grandparents, boyfriends or girlfriends of adolescents, and family acquaintances of the child who happen to be in the room. This situation needs to be handled carefully and, if possible, the IV procedure delayed until the parents are present. Parents may not extend a higher complement to a nurse than to allow him or her to care for their child. It is a tenuous privilege and one that parents evaluate constantly. Handle parents diplomatically to ensure a positive outcome.

Developmental Tasks

When children are allowed to rank their concerns in the hospital, they rank getting hurt, sharp things, and "getting a shot," at the top of the list. Venipuncture involves pain and sharp things, and the insertion is similar to getting a shot. Children deal with painful procedures differently than do adults, and their ability to cope is tempered with their perception of the situation and their ability to manage the situation.

TAKE HOME POINTS

- Concerns of children related to IV therapy are fairly consistent, regardless of developmental level.
- Children cope differently.

Developmental Tasks of Children Important to IV Therapy

Infant	
Developmental tasks	Trust vs. mistrust. The child is totally dependent on others and must learn that those entrusted with his or her care will provide everything. The child also develops gross motor and fine motor tasks and learns to pick up small things and bring them to the mouth for investigation.
Fears	Fears include falling, discomfort, needs not being met, and abandonment.
Responses to IV therapy	If the infant is a "graduate" of the neonatal intensive care unit, he or she will remember the IV process and start to resist by crying and displaying resistive movements the minute the child sees someone poised to do the venipuncture. The child cries and uses arm and leg movements to resist the procedure. He or she responds to soothing voices and *en face* positions and will watch an adult make faces at him or her.
Preparation of the child	Avoid feeding the child immediately before procedure. Pacifiers can be immensely comforting to babies in stressful situations. Babies must be kept warm during the procedure, and they do not like bright lights in their face but are fascinated with lights from a flashlight dancing across the ceiling. Keeping the bright light to a minimum will keep him or her happier. Babies like mobiles and being cuddled; they also like being rocked gently in a caregiver's arms.
Family	Parents will want to accompany the baby. Parents properly seated out of the way can provide great support to the infant, if they choose to be there. Family members should **not** restrain the child or participate directly in the venipuncture process.
Safety	The child's dominant hand or sucking fingers should be avoided in venipuncture efforts. A mobile tray or Mayo stand should be available to "set up" the venipuncture supplies and catch the little protective tips, papers, and other trash generated during the venipuncture process. The airway should be protected by holding the infant upright (holder's arm under baby's shoulders). Be sure to carefully monitor the child's color and respirations. Secure the site with a catheter securement system (e.g., Statlock). The site should be visible after dressing. Splints and restraint devices are sometimes used to protect the IV from inquisitive little fingers. These children should not be left by themselves on any surface, nor should the practitioner turn away from the infant without having a hand on the child.

Continued

Developmental Tasks of Children Important to IV Therapy–cont'd

Toddler

Developmental tasks	Autonomy vs. shame and doubt. This child enjoys rituals and has little concept of past or future. This phase is a highly negative stage, as the child masters his or her own body and the world around him or her. The child may start to see aggressive behavior. The child has many fantasies, enjoys new motor skills, and can indicate what he or she wants—even if the child cannot name it—by pointing.
Fears	Fears include injury, separation from the caregiver, loss of objects of comfort, being alone, and lack of ritual.
Responses to IV therapy	The child gains comfort from the parent's voice, even if the parent is not in view. The child attempts to bargain to avoid procedures (e.g., running away, getting involved in television, games). The child uses regressive behavior to try and stop venipuncture, such as screaming, loud crying, and so forth. Foot IVs on this group of patients is contraindicated; they are walking.
Preparation of the child	Prepare the child right before the venipuncture. Use simple terms and a calm, firm voice. Do not give this child choices when he or she does not have any, such as the common statement, "We're going to go do your IV now, okay?" What if the child says "no?" The battle now begins. Favorite toys or blankets may provide comfort to this child.
Family involvement	The child will be comforted by the parent's voice if the parent chooses to be in the room during venipuncture. If the parent does **not** want to be present, bring a picture of one of the parents with the child to the treatment room. Grandparents may be hurt by the child's gyrations and kicking, and the grandparents may have little patience for the toddler's acting-out behavior.
Safety	Restraining this child may require more than one method, such as an assistant and a sheet for a mummy restraint. A secure anchoring system is an absolute must for children in this age group. All IV connections should be taped. Be sure to secure IV sites and tubings so the child can play without tangling IV tubings in toy wheels or other moving parts. The pump should be completely out of the child's reach because a child in this age group has been well-educated on computers. Pump manipulations should be performed out of the child's direct vision. He or she can mimic observed behaviors accurately (e.g., setting a pump). Remember, this child views the IV pump as a toy and as the child's personal toy. He or she can also jump vigorously on the mattress; thus a frame over the crib is an important way of protecting this child from bouncing or climbing out of the crib.

Preschool

Developmental tasks	This child fears mutilation but is also interested in medical processes and is able to follow directions. Preschoolers have magical thinking and can, for example, imitate nursery rhyme characters as the IV is being put in and not even realize the IV is being placed.
Fears	Fears include bodily injury, loss of control, being in the dark, and being alone.

Developmental Tasks of Children Important to IV Therapy—cont'd

Preschool—cont'd

Responses to IV therapy	This child is curious about the IV but will, with reminders, avoid touching the IV site. These children derive comfort from having action figure toys (e.g., Barbie, soldier toys) accompany them to the treatment room. Cuddly toys such as teddy bears and other plush toys are also a great comfort to the preschool child.
Preparation of the child	Privacy is important. This child can understand simple explanations. The reason for the IV should be explained to the child so he or she connects the IV with getting well and feeling better. Although he or she may put up a brave front initially, this facade can crumble in the middle of the procedure; thus an assistant should always be available for IV placement. If he or she cannot cooperate at all, this child would do better with a small amount of sedation. If the facility has child-life specialists, this instance is definitely a time to use their skill in distraction. Encouraging the child to play the Big Bad Wolf, for example, and blowing away the IV, they huff and puff and huff and puff, and it works well. The child gets so involved with the rhythm of the rhyme that he or she forgets about the IV. Another idea is to let them sing a song that they like, a tune that has a soothing lyric. The louder they sing, the better. The nurse should praise and reward the child's cooperation lavishly, especially the first time he or she gets an IV. If not rewarded the first time, he or she will be resistive and hard to manage each time a new IV is needed.
Family role	This child may be more cooperative if the parent is not obvious. The parent should, however, provide comfort after the procedure. If the child "loses it" during the procedure, parents can sometimes be so mortified that they try to discipline the child instead of comfort him or her. This instance is not the time for discipline. The child should not associate venipuncture or any procedure with punitive consequences. If the child is simply too afraid to cooperate at all, the parent may want to leave the procedure room. The family should be encouraged to provide a reward that is specific for the child.
Safety	This child will probably need restraints, even if only minimal. Give the child enough time to bond with the person performing venipuncture. Reassure the child, if he or she becomes resistive, that hurting him or her is not intended. Prepare supplies ahead of time and keep them out of sight until the child is positioned, comfortable, and psychologically under control. Small bits and pieces of the venipuncture supplies should be out of the reach of this child. This child may go to preschool and is probably more savvy with a computer than is the nurse. Pumps and other controllers should not be within the reach of the child. Even the "lock-out" switch on the back of the pump is not too hard for these astute children to figure out. Be sure to check the patient-controlled analgesia (PCA) settings frequently; the child is also capable of reprogramming these devices.

Continued

Developmental Tasks of Children Important to IV Therapy—cont'd

School age

Developmental tasks	This child has a sense of industry, understands the relationship between illness and treatment in concrete terms, and is aware of danger. The child can follow directions without frequent reminders and struggles between mastery and failure; thus any success should be complimented. Because peer group recognition is important, visits to the hospital of his or her friends should be sanctioned and supported. Telephone conversations are also important and should not be interrupted if at all possible.
Fears	Fears include death, mutilation, loss of control, and the inability to live up to the expectations of others.
Responses to IV therapy	Help the child to be in control. Let him or her set the pace of venipuncture by choosing the arm to have the IV. This child may deny the need for the IV by denying he or she is ill because of fear of death. The child may not want the parent present during venipuncture. If this desire is a problem for the parent, communicate with the parent the importance of the child maintaining some control over the environment. If the child loses this battle, he or she has lost control of the situation.
Preparation of the child	This child does well with preparation in advance of the venipuncture, even several hours. Explain in detail how venipuncture is done; he or she may want to know. Allow the child to help in body positioning if he or she is able. The assistant is in stand-by mode "to help the child if he needs it." The assistant is also important in distracting this child as much as possible. Reassure this child that crying is OK and that he or she will have time to regain composure, if necessary, after the procedure is completed. Television provides a great distraction.
Family role	Let the child chose whether the parent is present. Prepare the child and parent together. The period between one IV and the next can sometimes be used for a shower, time away from the pediatric unit, or other enjoyable activities that the family can share.
Safety	Playfulness in this group and his or her denial of being ill can lead to bravado with IV equipment that can cause accidents or injuries. Allow this child as much mobility as possible. **Remind** the child gently about safety with IV equipment and to avoid adjusting the IV pump or PCA settings. Children in this group are even more acquainted with computers than are preschool children and are fully capable of reprogramming an IV pump. Turn the pump away from the child's field of vision for adjustments.

Adolescents

Developmental tasks	This child has a sense of identity, hovers between independence and dependence, and questions authority figures. A strong need exists for privacy. The child is able to understand abstract ideas and to consider alternatives. Peer acceptance is important.
Fears	Fears include loss of control, altered body image, and separation from peers.
Responses to IV therapy	The adolescent is hyperresponsive to pain, regresses to a lower developmental stage of behavior, and is resistant to authority figures and parents. Noncompliance with medication and treatment plan may be present. Illness is a threat to body integrity; disease means ugliness. The adolescent may pull out IVs as part of the denial process or as a means of getting attention.

Developmental Tasks of Children Important to IV Therapy—cont'd

Adolescents—cont'd

Preparation of the child	Offer choices. Most of these children are able to back up a solid "**no**." Provide as much advance notice as possible. Allow him or her to ask questions and make known his or her desires and concerns about the procedure.
Family role	Make sure the parent is present during explanations. Adolescents may not listen to everything that is said. Encourage family members to support the adolescent's reasonable decisions. Assure the family that the adolescent needs to direct his or her own care.
Safety	Adolescents love to "clown around" and may endanger the IV site. Teach the adolescent to report observations about the IV promptly. Check the pump rates frequently; adolescents can figure out how to reset rates, among other things. This child may insist on a boyfriend or girlfriend being present during procedures. As
long	as visitors are properly prepared, there is no reason they cannot be seated on the opposite side of the bed to provide attention and distraction to the adolescent patient.

Adapted from Infusion Therapy in Clinical Practice, 2001.

What You DO

Consider the child's chronologic age and developmental stage when developing an IV plan of care. Make all attempts to anticipate and minimize stress because this can adversely affect the venipuncture process. A stressed child releases epinephrine when afraid, causing vasoconstriction. Before beginning the insertion procedure, communicate with the parents or caregivers to determine their roles. Safety is an important consideration in IV care. The child must be protected, based on his or her development capabilities, from hazards related to IV therapy.

Physical comfort and ambient temperatures and lighting must be considered, especially when providing IV care to premature infants.

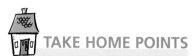

TAKE HOME POINTS

Children's veins are smaller, shorter, and more delicate than those of adults.

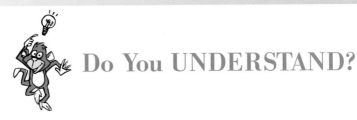

Do You UNDERSTAND?

DIRECTIONS: **Match the developmental stage in Column A with the best nursing approach in Column B.**

Column A

1. _____ Infant
2. _____ Toddler
3. _____ Preschooler
4. _____ School-age child
5. _____ Adolescent

Column B

a. This child might appreciate having a boyfriend or girlfriend present during venipuncture.
b. This child should not be offered choices.
c. An IV should not be placed in this child's sucking fingers.
d. This child likes to have the IV process explained.
e. This child may need extra observation to prevent reckless behavior with the IV site or equipment.

DIRECTIONS: **Identify the following statement as *true* (T) or *false* (F).**

6. _____ Parents should be allowed to participate actively in the actual IV placement process.

DIRECTIONS: **Select the best answer from the options provided.**

7. _____ Select the child who should not have his or her telephone conversations interrupted to place an IV.

   a. Toddler   c. School-age child
   b. Preschooler   d. Adolescent

8. _____ Keeping the "bits and pieces" away from which group of children is a most important safety consideration?

   a. Infant   c. School-age child
   b. Preschooler   d. Adolescent

9. _____ Cold stress is a hazard for small babies and complicates IV placement in babies because:

 a. They can experience vasoconstriction.

 b. They begin to burn brown-fat stores.

 c. The child becomes acidotic as a result of fat metabolism.

 d. All of the above are true.

10. _____ Grandma Kelly is staying with Baby Bryan in the hospital while her daughter works. Her daughter must work because she has the insurance coverage for herself and her children. The older children are in school, and Grandma and Mom trade places after work, with Grandma going home to care for the older children and Mom staying with Baby Bryan at night. This arrangement has been particularly stressful for the family. Baby Bryan now needs an IV after a day of fitful crying and outbursts. Grandma insists on accompanying Baby Bryan to the treatment room for his IV placement. What is the best way to handle this situation?

 a. Invite Grandma to take a break and have a cup of coffee.

 b. Insist that Grandma wait in the playroom.

 c. Tell Grandma that if she would like to take a break, she can do so.

 d. Tell Grandma that the IV can be restarted later, and allow her to spend some unencumbered moments with this child, holding and rocking him in the rocking chair.

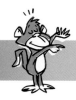

What IS the Insertion Process?

Cannulating pediatric veins is difficult. When the child is ill or injured, the task is even more difficult. Inserting a peripheral IV into a pediatric patient is challenging and requires practice to become comfortable and proficient.

Answers: 9. d: Brown-fat metabolism produces ketones, which lead to acidosis and vasoconstriction; **10. d:** This caregiver has had an exhausting day with this child and has an even more stressful time awaiting her when she returns home to care for the older children. A respite would be good for her and even better for Baby Bryan.

What You NEED TO KNOW

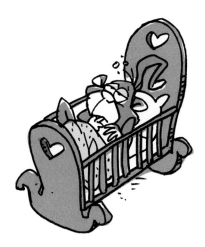

Assuming that an order has been written for an IV or that an order exists implicating the need for an IV, the allergies and other mitigating circumstances for pediatric IV therapy must be addressed. Before beginning the venipuncture procedure, careful consideration to the developmental needs of the child should be made. For example, does the baby suck his or her thumb or fingers for comfort? Does the child need a special toy or stuffed animal for comfort during stressful procedures? Does the older child understand how the IV will help him or her get well or feel better? Is the IV the only way or the best way to address the child's medicinal needs? These issues should be reviewed regularly with the medical staff, especially as the number of possible IV sites declines.

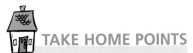

TAKE HOME POINTS

Holding the child is the most important job in the venipuncture process.

Assistance for holding the child (no parents please) must be procured. The roles of the inserter and the holder must be clearly defined and agreed to before the child or the parent is involved. The inserter should be capable of successfully inserting the IV in one attempt. The holder should be familiar with the venipuncture process so that skillful assistance can be provided to the inserter when necessary without compromising the venipuncture process or releasing the child. The holder should be "in tune" with the inserter and follow the lead of the inserter. No friction should exist between the inserter and the holder. Additionally, the holder should be able to gently restrain the child's movements and keep the child psychologically secure so the venipuncture can proceed in an expeditious manner. The holder will also address any questions from the parent if present (see color plate 19).

Job Description of the Child Holder

- If the child requires cardiac monitoring or pulse oximetry, monitor this data.
- The needs of the child and the inserter should be anticipated.
- The holder should be capable of soothing the child and the parent.
- The holder should be strong enough to secure the limb selected for the IV in an absolutely still position to enhance the likelihood of successful venipuncture.
- During the dressing portion of IV insertion, the holder and inserter must work in concert with each other to ensure that the dressing is applied securely to the IV site and that the splint is applied without pressure to the child's limb.

- The holder should also direct the parents so their presence is optimal to successful venipuncture.
- If the parent is present during the insertion procedure, keep him or her informed of progress, plans, and options as the procedure progresses.
- The parents should be educated about how best to protect the site and help it last longer. If the child is old enough, the child can be advised as to the best way to protect his or her new IV.
- It helps to keep stickers in the treatment room to reward the child for his or her cooperation. This decoration process can begin to help the child accept this process and make it more palatable.

What You DO

Prepare the room in which the venipuncture will take place. It is important to the security and psychologic comfort of the other children in the nursing unit not to hear another child screaming in panic.

The ambient temperature must be kept reasonably warm for young children. If the room temperature is not adjustable, ancillary sources of heat— blankets and towels— should be used, and infant heel warmers are helpful and just the right size for a child.

Before the patient's arrival to the insertion room, set up the venipuncture site to allow efficient progress from one step of the venipuncture process to the next. All the supplies and equipment for venipuncture should be assembled on a stand or table. This assembly area should be a different surface than that on which the child will be placed. With the exception of the largest of children, a 24-gauge catheter is common for pediatric patients. On rare occasions, a 22-gauge catheter may be used and, with adolescent children, even a 20-gauge catheter. Place several catheters on the tray. Include a primed extension set and a catheter-stabilization mechanism. Cover the tray. Obvious supplies are intimidating and stressful to the child. Even the youngest child will learn with each successive IV placement to identify venipuncture equipment. The tray should be positioned with easy access for the inserting nurse but at a safe distance from the child. In addition to the IV equipment, some suggestions for an IV "toolbox" include:

- Hemostat for loosening tubing connections
- Scissors for cutting tape (never to be used around an IV site; they may cut off a little finger)

TAKE HOME POINTS

Without an effective holder, the child might get loose and resist the venipuncture process.

TAKE HOME POINTS

If the child has an infection, is in traction, or has heavy casts or orthopedic appliances, the IV may need to be started in his or her room.

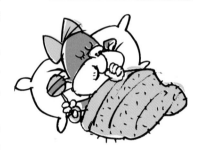

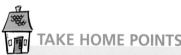

TAKE HOME POINTS

The child's veins become vasoconstricted when he or she gets cold.

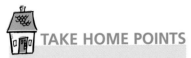

TAKE HOME POINTS

Do not keep tape in toolbox; it will harbor microbes.

- Mag-Light flashlight
- Sharpie marker for dating dressings
- IV drug book
- Hospital IV policy and pediatric IV policies
- Post-It Notes for messages to physicians
- Stickers for decorating new IV sites

Make sure adequate lighting is available in the room, as well as a Mag-Light or otoscope. The child's additional needs should be considered (e.g., pulse oximetry, suction, oxygen, electrocardiogram monitoring) and provided for. Position the trash can so that the inserting nurse can dispose of all paper, as well as small bits and pieces during the insertion procedure, to prevent the child from having access to anything. A sharps disposal system should be in reach of the inserting nurse. The safety of the parent should also be considered when setting up the treatment room. Parents should have a chair in which to sit and a way to exit quickly if needed.

Determining Parental Involvement

Discuss the parents' involvement with them before talking to the child. Good parental involvement, if the parent or parents wish to be included in this process, starts with good information. Excluding the parents should be a mutual decision between the parents and the nurse. The nurse should realize that excluding the parents might increase the child's anxiety momentarily and increase the burden on the holder to keep the child distracted, relaxed, and cooperative. The parent should never be made to feel that his or her parenting is below standard if he or she chooses not to accompany the child. If the family is a blended family, careful consideration of who accompanies the child should be worked out with all the adults, ahead of time. The best interests of the child should be clearly focused for everyone involved in his or her care. The parents should be assured that no matter what the behavior of their child is during the venipuncture procedure, it is not unique and will not be outrageous to the nursing staff, no matter how noisy it becomes. If a parent seems reluctant to be involved, he or she would probably appreciate the suggestion to take a much-needed break.

Making the decision about whether the parents should accompany the child to the treatment room is not to be taken lightly. This decision has legal implications. Make sure to find out who has the legal guardianship of the child. Do not make this part of the decision-making process obvious to the nonbiologic members in a blended family. Although determining legal

TAKE HOME POINTS

The parent should be educated about the basic process and what is expected of them to enhance the venipuncture process.

responsibility is important, people close to the patient may be offended if excluded. If the child is a ward of the state, make sure the responsible guardian is notified before procedures are undertaken.

Patient Preparation

Educate the child honestly and simply about the IV procedure based on their developmental stage. Discussion during the procedure should be minimal, and a "debriefing" should follow the procedure to allow the child to ventilate and feel less violated and more in control. The child's behavior should never be categorized as good or bad. A child might believe that illness is punishment for bad behavior and that good behavior has no reward other than painful procedures. Be careful of certain phrases and words that the child, depending on his or her age and stage of development, can misinterpret. A toddler might envision a tree branch in his or her skin if the nurse tells the child that he or she will get a small "stick." Instead, an alternative might be that the catheter is going to be put "under your skin." Adolescents are particularly uncomfortable when professionals talk "around" them without being involved in the conversation. Limit setting is particularly important in performing venipuncture on children. Telling them, "It's OK to cry, but don't move the arm" lets the child and the parent know exactly what behavior is acceptable, and the parent can remind the child to cooperate. If the parent is not in the room, the holder can remind the child, as necessary, especially if the child does not know the person who is placing the IV. Medical play, especially after the procedure, allows the child to examine the equipment used for the IV procedure and to reduce the effect of unrealistic fears.

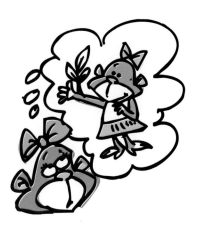

Pain Management

This area is an important facet of pediatric IV care. Children have long memories of "owwies" and are intolerant of any discomfort when they are ill. There are many ways to minimize pain in pediatric IV therapy. Some of these techniques are listed here. Each of these methods has advantages for children and can be used in combination or progression as necessary to help the child. The child's own imagination can be a powerful tool to help prevent discomfort during venipuncture.

- Puppetry. Using puppets or toys that are manipulated as puppets allows the child to "talk out" his or her fears and needs in a nonthreatening manner. The feel of plush toys is also comforting to a child. Brushing it against the child's skin has a calming effect on the child.

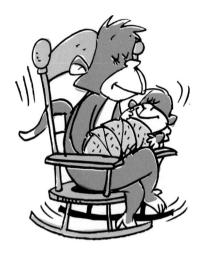

- Imagery. Helping the child envision a special place or event is also calming during the procedure. Continuing the imagery will distract the child during the venipuncture process. One favorite image among toddlers and preschoolers is the Big Bad Wolf—and they huff and puff and blow the IV away. If the holder is really good, the child gets so engrossed in the imagery, he or she forgets about the IV. Singing can also help the child forget about what the inserter is doing. Any of the nursery rhyme songs are wonderful and easy for the child to imagine.

- Distraction and rocking. This technique is comforting to infants. A soothing voice, combined with gentle rocking movements via the holder, can help the child relax. *En face* positions distract the infant so well that he or she may drift off to sleep.

- Inducement. This technique can be an effective tool to secure cooperation. Inducement works well with some older children, especially for the child who has been in the hospital for a lengthy period. The child can be offered a tempting reward for his or her cooperation. Do not use the parents' presence as a bribe for cooperation. The child should be able to count on his or her parents' presence whenever needed. Inducement items might include computer game time, extra time in the playroom, art supplies, riding in the wagon with the nurse pulling it, popsicles, ice cream, playing with some of the supplies for venipuncture (e.g., syringes without needles), or any combination of these items.

- Anesthetic creams and sedation. Pain management is important in pediatric IV therapy. Children have **no** tolerance for physical discomfort of any kind. Anesthetic creams such as eutectic mixture of local anesthetics (EMLA) or ELA-max (see Chapter 2) can help prevent physical discomfort; but do not expect a silent IV start. The psychologic discomfort of being restrained may be more than the child can tolerate. Occasionally, sedation with Benadryl, choral hydrate, or other pharmaceutical drugs may be required to ease both physical and psychologic discomfort (if medically appropriate and with a physician's order).

Achieving Cooperation

It is important that the child feels the security of a solid front between the nursing staff and the parents. He or she will feel more comfortable and be more malleable during procedures if the child believes there are no alternatives to the procedure. Be careful not to give the child choices when he or she has none. Do not ask the child not to protest the venipuncture process; rather, ask for only a small amount of cooperation, such as not moving the arm. Integrate inducements that are based on developmental stage into the

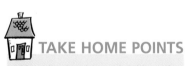

TAKE HOME POINTS

Although a head-injured child may be highly combative, it is medically inappropriate to use sedation.

procedure explanation. Any cooperation the child is able to provide should be rewarded with something the child would like to have.

Patient Positioning

Unless the child has a fever, the only appendage that should be free is the one in which the IV is to be inserted. The head should be supported and elevated because infants and young children tend to vomit when stressed (see color plate 20). It is easier for the holder to assist the inserter when the baby is swaddled in a light blanket (see color plate 21). The holder should offer soothing verbal coaching to the child and ensure that his or her stress level is minimized. The child should **never** be left unattended on any surface. If the nurse must turn away from the child, he or she should grasp an arm or leg of the child for safety, meaning that the nurse should never be more than an arm's length away from the child. Holding an older child is even more of a challenge. Older children are much more capable than are their younger counterparts of avoiding venipuncture. Additional help to hold thrashing legs and feet may be needed. A preadolescent child who refuses to cooperate should be given as much room and time as he or she needs to regain composure and rethink the need for the IV. This instance is definitely one in which the parent can assist in the venipuncture process. An adolescent who ardently refuses to cooperate should **not** be physically restrained by the nursing staff. Solicit the parent's assistance in convincing the child to allow the IV placement or rethink the need for the IV.

Venipuncture Procedure

Wash hands and put on gloves.

- **Step 1: Vein selection:** Finding the best vein for the IV involves skill and careful assessment. All potential vein sites in all four extremities should be assessed, unless one arm or leg is not to be used for some reason. If possible, offering the dehydrated child some oral fluids can improve vein size by expanding the circulating volume. If oral fluids are not a possibility, then warming the child can also cause an artificial vasodilatation to enhance venipuncture efforts. Transillumination of veins using a Mag-Light flashlight or an otoscope works well in small babies, dark-skinned children, or plump toddlers, as well as visualizing deeper veins. By shining the light through the child's arm or hand, the venous network is easily visualized as a black line against a red background (see color plate 22). This process is inexpensive, works well, and is interesting to the child. Rubbing the child's skin with a wet alcohol or saline wipe will help the veins become more visible in a room lighted by fluorescent lights. The use of small heel warmers

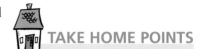

TAKE HOME POINTS

- A crying child may not be upset about the venipuncture process. He or she may not like being without his parental caregiver; he or she may be cold, wet, or hungry; or he or she may not like the treatment room.
- Children experience vasoconstriction quickly because they get upset quickly; they must be kept calm and comfortable.

to dilate tiny foot veins may help when the foot is involved. When using a tourniquet, do not tie too tightly; and do not leave a tourniquet tied longer than 1 minute at a time. Baby veins are delicate and can bleed with a tight tourniquet. Release the tourniquet, let the arm rest while continuing to assess the veins, and then reapply it. Both arms should be checked carefully by palpation, inspection, and transillumination. This method takes time, and the parent, if present, should understand that this procedure is an important part of finding the "right" vein (see color plate 23). Several processes may need to be used, such as transillumination and heat, to locate the appropriate vein. The vein selection process may take 30 minutes or longer to fully assess all venous possibilities. The harder this process becomes, the more consideration should be focused on IV alternatives or central venous access devices. Do not choose venous sites in feet of walking babies or children. Be careful of veins in the wrist joint if movement is a problem and if the possibility of nicking an artery is present. Rubber bands placed on the infant's head are commonly used to promote vein dilation when using a scalp vein. Place the infant such that his or her head is lower than the rest of the body, which will usually cause crying. The position and crying enhance vein dilation. Scalp veins should be used as a last resort.

The best vein is defined as one that is palpable, fills readily after being depressed, and is long enough to allow **full** insertion of the IV catheter. The vein should be located in an area that allows comfortable movement for the child.

TAKE HOME POINTS

Check all possible locations of veins before the best vein is selected.

- Step 2: Skin preparation: Select the proper skin antiseptic according to facility protocol. Apply a tourniquet and evaluate the venous selection one more time and then release. Clean the site (see Chapter 2). Let all preparing agents dry. Preparation pads can be used to mark the location of the vein after preparing simply by laying the pad on the child's skin with the tip "marking the spot." This practice helps prevent the practitioner from violating the "no-touch" principle after preparing the skin. Apply the tourniquet.

TAKE HOME POINTS

Be sure to inquire whether the facility policy requires alcohol or povidone iodine used as a preparation for babies.

- Step 3: Vein stabilization: Proper vein stabilization is a key ingredient to successful venipuncture. Taping the arm to a board before the venipuncture process is initiated will give support to the hand or arm so the nurse can apply traction to the vein (see color plate 24). With small infants or older cooperative children, bringing the fingers down toward the inner arm will make the arm more stable, enabling application of sufficient traction to the vein for proper stabilization (see color plate 25). With larger infants, this technique may not be possible because they are capable of active and effective resistance.

TAKE HOME POINTS

The vein should be stabilized until the catheter is completely inserted.

- Step 4: Insertion: The angle of approach is different in pediatrics—it should be shallow (10 to 20 degrees). Using an indirect approach makes venipuncture easier in young children who usually get highly animated after the stylet pierces the skin. However, whether the skin is pierced directly over the vein or parallel to the vein is a judgment call of the nurse who is inserting the IV and the abilities of the holder. The catheter and stylet are advanced together slowly until a blood return is observed. The flashback of blood may be slow and small in quantity. If a blood return is not immediately seen, wait a second or two, or place a warm compress over the vein to promote a flashback, or both. The needle needs to be advanced only slightly to ensure that the tip of the catheter is in the lumen of the vein. Retract the stylet slightly into the catheter hooding it, and then continue advancing until the catheter hub is at the skin line. Release the tourniquet. Remember to keep an eye on the vein; do not be distracted. Pediatric IV catheters are only $^1/_2$- to $^3/_4$-inches long, and any movement can displace the catheter out of the vein. If resistance is met while advancing the catheter, remove the stylet, attach a primed extension set, and (using a saline-filled 3-cc syringe and while slowly injecting saline) advance the catheter into the vein. This technique is called floating the catheter in. No swelling should be noted at the catheter tip or insertion site during this process. If swelling is noted, immediately stop the insertion process and discontinue the IV. (See Chapter 2.)

  Number of attempts: Although the Infusion Nursing Society (INS) recommends only two attempts per nurse, many pediatric facilities allow only one. Limiting the number of unsuccessful attempts and allowing the child rest time between series of attempts is important. Considering other forms of IV therapy or other medicinal alternatives may also be necessary.

- Step 5: Catheter stabilization: Stabilizing a catheter is an important and challenging process with the pediatric patient. Once the hub of the catheter is fully inserted to the skin line, with the stylet still in place, apply the dressing according to facility policy. The insertion site should be visible for frequent observation. After the dressing is applied, place a sterile gauze under the hub (to catch any blood that may leak from the hub). Then, while applying slight pressure on the vein above the catheter tip with a finger, remove the stylet and apply the primed extension set to the hub. Flush the catheter and observe for swelling at the catheter tip. Motion is generally the action that dislodges IVs in the pediatric patient; stabilization and protective devices prevent these dislodgments. Examples are Statlock or IV House (see color plates 26, 27, and 28).

TAKE HOME POINTS

The traction on the vein is maintained throughout the venipuncture process.

TAKE HOME POINTS

Accuracy is important in most pediatric settings because the total number of IV attempts per day may be limited.

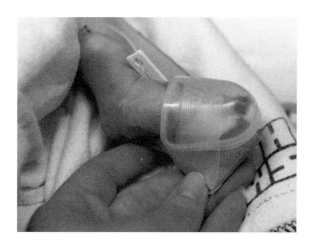

Without proper stabilization, even the tiniest baby can "rub out" an IV. The tubing connections should be padded to protect the child's skin from cuts and tears by the tubing. One piece of gauze under the hub of the catheter helps protect the child's skin from cuts and irritation. The INS recommends a splint to support the IV site if the catheter is located through or near a joint. A splint also helps prevent motion of the limb and stress to the catheter site (see color plate 27). Careful placement of the extension set and IV tubing will prevent potential entanglement of the tubing in wheeled toys and other play activities. Apply decorative stickers and provide a reward and verbal praise to the child. Date the dressing, indicate the gauge of the catheter, and include initials.

Caring for the IV

Most pediatric facilities require that the sites are checked at least hourly to ensure patency and lack of complications. Steps for making the pediatric IV last longer include:

- Maintaining the stabilization system
- Elevating the child's limb on towels or blankets
- Preventing vein irritations through proper dilution of medicines
- Instructing the parents in proper care of the site and encouraging them to distract the child's attention away from the IV
- Frequent, proper flushing and appropriate disconnecting procedures

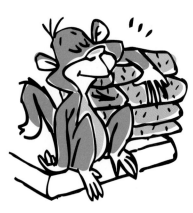

In children over 28 days of age, saline is just as effective as is heparin in maintaining catheter patency, without the worries of thrombocytopenia. In very small infants, a membrane filter can significantly reduce the particulates delivered to the child's pulmonary bed. Without filtration, the particulates can cause capillary occlusion, which may produce tissue anoxia, cell death, and an inflammatory reaction. Particles small enough to bypass the lung capillaries may cause similar pathologic lesions in the eye, brain, kidneys, liver, or spleen. At the infusion site, these particles may cause local inflammatory reactions.

Peripheral venous catheters may be left in place until IV therapy is complete, unless a complication occurs (as recommended by the Centers for Disease Control and Prevention [CDC]). Know the institution policy for catheter rotation. All pediatric IV solutions and medications should be delivered by an electronic pump with free flow protection to prevent fluid overload or speed shock. Metered volume chamber sets (e.g., Buretrol) (see Chapter 1) assist in limiting the amount of fluid that can be delivered to the child to prevent sudden circulatory overload. Children are at increased risk for fluid overload. Fluid overload is especially serious in the infant and small child.

Detecting Problems with the IV

The most common problem encountered with pediatric IVs is infiltration (for more information, see Chapter 3) (see color plate 29). This problem exists because of the increased activity level of children. Even children with a great deal of adipose tissue will show tissue distention and tightness with infiltration. Comparing one limb with the other is an excellent technique to detect beginning infiltration. Checking the site with a flashlight will help identify beginning phlebitis, noted as a pink line along the vein tract. Pay particular attention when the child is receiving irritant or vesicant medications. Catheter occlusion is another problem encountered in pediatrics. (For more information, see Chapter 3.) This problem occurs because of the small catheter gauge size and the small vein size of the child. Occluded peripheral catheters are removed and replaced if necessary. Phlebitis occurs less often in children under 10 years of age AND then begins to increase to adult levels as the child's age increases.

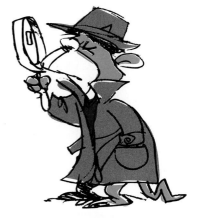

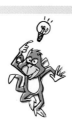

Do You UNDERSTAND?

DIRECTIONS: Complete the crossword puzzle by answering the questions related to preparing the room in which the venipuncture will take place.

Across:

2. What must be kept reasonably warm for young children *(2 words, no space)*?
4. On what should supplies be assembled?
5. What needs to be near the inserting nurse *(2 words, no space)*?

Down:

1. What will prevent a child from playing with disposable paper items *(2 words, no space)*?
3. What is used to provide light for selecting a vein?

DIRECTIONS: Unscramble the words that describe ways to minimize pain during pediatric IV therapy.

1. _____ (tupreppy)

2. _____   _____
_____ (ctridaston nda korcgin)

3. _____ (decinumten)

4. _____   _____
_____   _____ (nitashetce mceras nda stedaino)

DIRECTIONS: Identify the following statements as *true* (**T**) or *false* (**F**).

5. _____ A crying child may not be upset about the venipuncture process.

6. _____ Children experience vasoconstriction slowly because they get upset quickly.

7. _____ Unless the child has a fever, the only appendage that should be free is the one in which the IV is to be inserted.

8. _____ The most important factor in decreasing the life of an IV catheter is catheter motion.

DIRECTIONS: Fill in the blanks to complete each statement.

9. The best vein is defined as one that is _____,

_____   _____ after being

depressed, and is _____   _____

to allow **complete** insertion of the IV catheter.

10. The pediatric insertion angle is _____

than that of adult insertions.

DIRECTIONS: **Select the best answer.**

11. _____ A reasonable pattern of checking a pediatric IV should be:
   a. Every 1 to 2 hours
   b. Every 4 hours
   c. In accordance with facility policy
   d. Both a and c
   e. None of the above

12. _____ How many attempts should a nurse make to start or restart an IV?
   a. One
   b. Two
   c. Four
   d. As many as it takes
   e. None of the above

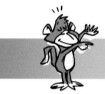

What IS a Pediatric Central Venous Catheter?

Types of CVCs are the same in the pediatric patient as those in the adult population (see Chapter 4 for in-depth information regarding CVCs).

What You NEED TO KNOW

CVCs selected for insertion are of smaller gauge than those of the adult patient. Insertion site option preferences are also different. Insertion sites are chosen according to the inserting physician's preference, safety issues, and accessibility.

Common Insertion Site Options

CATHETER TYPE	INSERTION SITES
STCVC	Subclavian veins, internal jugular veins, femoral veins (inferior vena cava)
Tunneled	Superior vena cava with chest exit site or inferior vena cava with the exit site on abdomen, thigh, or back
Implanted	Superior or inferior vena cava with port placed on chest, arm, or abdomen
PICC (infants)	Saphenous superficial temporal, external jugular, popliteal, axillary
PICC (children)	Same as adults (see Chapter 4)

What You DO

Because the gauge size is small, it is important to flush the CVC appropriately (see Chapter 4). Occlusion can occur more often in the pediatric population than the adult population. Flushing catheters requires different volumes than those required with adult CVCs.

Flushing Procedure for CVCs (Adapted from *Infusion Therapy in Clinical Practice*, 2001.)

	INTERMITTENT FLUSHING	AFTER BLOOD DRAW	MAINTENANCE
Nontunneled	3 ml 0.9% normal saline (NS), 1 ml heparinized saline* solution	5-10 ml NS, 1-3 ml heparinized saline solution	1-3 ml heparinized saline solution, every 8-24 hr
PICC	2-3 ml NS, 1-2 ml heparinized saline solution	5-10 ml NS, 1-2 ml heparinized saline solution	1-2 ml heparinized saline solution daily or twice a day
Tunneled (valved tip catheters need NS only)	3 ml NS, 2-5 ml heparinized saline solution	5-10 ml NS, 2-5 ml heparinized saline solution	2-5 ml heparinized saline solution daily to weekly
Implanted port	5 ml NS, 2 ml heparinized saline solution	5-10 ml NS, 5 ml heparinized saline solution	5 ml heparinized saline solution every 30 days

*The concentration of heparin in heparinized saline solution commonly used with central venous access ranges from 10 to 100 units/ml. The concentration used for flushing is determined by institution procedure. The solution should be benzyl-alcohol free. Solutions with benzyl-alcohol preservative should not be used with neonates weighing less than 1200 g (2.65 pounds).

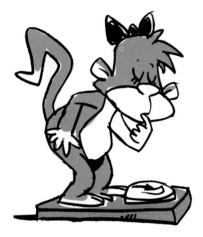

Routine CVC dressing changes for the pediatric patient should be weighed against the risk of dislodging the catheter. The CDC does not recommend routine dressing changes for the pediatric patient. Although chlorhexidine sponges are recommended for the pediatric patient's high risk of infection (such as those in the intensive care setting), they should not be used in neonates under age 7 days or of gestational age under 26 weeks (CDC recommendations).

Declotting CVCs depends on the type and gauge of the catheter plus the volume of all add-on devices that are present. The type of declotting agent depends on what is occluding the catheter (see Chapter 5). If using alteplase (Cath-Flo), the maximum dose is 0.4 mg/kg. Doses of alteplase are sent from pharmacy based on the patient's weight and do not factor in the type, size, and volume of the catheter and all of the add-ons. The nurse may need to dilute the alteplase with normal saline (0.9% sodium chloride) if the volume sent from the pharmacy is less than the volume of the catheter plus all add-on devices that are present. The nurse may need to discard a small part of the alteplase dose if the volume sent from the pharmacy is larger than the volume of the catheter plus all add-on devices that are present.

Dosing Table Examples

Patient >0.5 to <2.0 kg

Catheter Volume	Alteplase Dose/Volume
0.0-0.5 ml	0.2 mg/0.2 ml
>0.5-1.0 ml	0.2 mg/0.2 ml
>1.0 ml	0.2 mg/0.2 ml

Patient 2.0 to <5.0 kg

Catheter Volume	Alteplase Dose/Volume
0.0-0.5 ml	0.5 mg/0.5 mL
>0.5-1.0 ml	0.5 mg/0.5 mL
>1.0 ml	0.5 mg/0.5 mL

Patient 5.0 kg

Catheter Volume	Alteplase Dose/Volume
0.0-0.5 ml	0.5 mg/0.5 mL
>0.5-1.0 ml	1.0 mg/1.0 mL
>1.0 ml	2.0 mg/2.0 mL

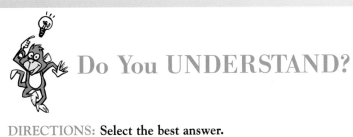

Do You UNDERSTAND?

DIRECTIONS: **Select the best answer.**

1. _____ The smaller-gauge catheters increase the incidence of which of the following problems:
    a. Phlebitis in children under age 10 years
    b. Occlusion
    c. Infiltration
    d. All of the above

DIRECTIONS: **Fill in the blanks to complete the statements.**

2. _____ _____ preservative

   should not be used with neonates weighing less than 1200 g (2.65 lb).

3. Routine CVC dressing changes for the pediatric patient should be

   weighed against the _____ ____

   _____ the catheter.

4. Declotting CVCs depends on the _____ and

   _____ of the catheter plus the _____

   of all add-on devices that are present.

7 Older Adult Patient

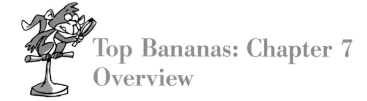

Top Bananas: Chapter 7 Overview

Who IS the Older Adult Patient?

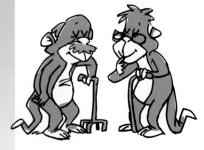

Older adults are a special patient population who have specific needs and requirements to ensure safe and successful intravenous (IV) care. The geriatric population is increasing and will continue to do so for the next 15 to 20 years. Statistics indicate that approximately 20% of the population is over the age of 65. By the year 2020 it is projected that number will increase to 27%. Additionally, individuals aged 85 to 100 years have dramatically increased as well.

To care for geriatric patients properly, the nurse must be informed about the normal physiologic changes that affect the skin, veins, immune system, liver, and kidneys. Most of the changes related to aging begin around age 60 and progresses slowly over the rest of a person's lifetime. Lack of awareness of the predictable physiologic system changes will increase the risk of complications and adverse effects of IV delivery. These occurrences cause excess trauma to an individual, may prolong hospitalization, and increase the overall cost of care.

What You NEED TO KNOW

Older adults are divided into three groups based on age: young-old (65 to 74 years), middle-old (75 to 84 years), and old-old (greater than 84 years). The body changes with age. None of these changes are diseases, and all are normal as related to aging. The changes described here are less significant in the young-old and the most significant in the old-old. Older adults may be more apprehensive about receiving IV therapy because of misconceptions about infusions. Many seniors believe that IVs are started only on critically ill people and may believe they are dying. Reassurance and education about current IV practice will help to relieve these fears.

Decreases in immunity begin around age 30, but these decreases become significant after age 60.

Skin Changes

The changes that will affect IV therapy practice occurring in the skin and tissues surrounding the veins begin at approximately 60 to 65 years of age. With the loss of collagen and subcutaneous fat associated with increased elastic tissue, the skin becomes increasingly transparent. The layers of the skin are thin, becoming more fragile and less elastic, which makes the skin prone to tearing, ulceration, or both. There is an actual loss of cells in the epidermis and dermis that will create less resistance to an IV catheter passing through the skin. The loss of subcutaneous tissue along the hands, forearms, and upper arms makes veins less stable and creates a tendency for them to move more freely (roll) under the skin. The number of nerve endings in the skin decrease with age. The older adult patient may not be able to feel pain and pressure as acutely as would a younger adult, making them less aware of the early signs of the complication of infiltration.

 TAKE HOME POINTS

If an individual has spent excess time exposed to sunlight, the epidermis will be toughened or damaged (or both) and may have a leathery texture.

Vein Changes

The vein wall changes in a number of ways. The adventitia has more connective tissue and the media has less smooth muscle (see Chapter 2 for more information). These changes make the vein wall thicker and the vein less elastic. Loss of elasticity inhibits the vein's ability to distend as readily. With advancing age, the connective tissue is reabsorbed, and the vein is weakened, making it much more easily torn by the introduction of a catheter. This change makes older adults more prone to subcutaneous bleeding. Throughout the aging process, small veins and capillaries will become thinner and more fragile, causing them to rupture on puncture. Damage to the subclavian vein or the vena cava in the old-old can have catastrophic consequences, with serious intrathoracic hemorrhage. In addition, valves in the peripheral veins will become less flexible and efficient with aging.

Physiologic Changes

Liver: As a person ages, the liver reduces to almost one third of its original size. This lessened mass creates an altered function. There is a reduction in the production of oxidizing enzymes for drug metabolism. Additionally, the amount of protein synthesis will decrease, resulting in a lower amount of blood albumin. Both of these changes will affect drug levels in the body. The reduction in oxidation of enzymes will create a prolonged drug level in the bloodstream. The projected drug half-life will be lengthened. The lack of protein-binding sites in the plasma will create more free drug in the blood.

Kidney: The loss of functioning nephrons begins gradually at approximately 40 years of age. Over the next 50 years (until age 90), as many as 50% of an individual's original nephrons may be lost, causing the remaining nephrons to have a reduced rate of filtration (some by as much as 50%). The estimated decline in filtration will eventually create a potential filtration rate of 60 to 70 cc per minute from an original rate of 120 cc per minute. The loss of functioning nephrons in the kidneys will reduce the ability to handle IV fluids infused into the body. The diminished filtration rate of the remaining nephrons will also affect the body's ability to properly handle extra fluids infused and cause a "back-up" or "build-up" of fluid in the body. This condition is often seen clinically as pulmonary edema or circulatory overload. Additionally, because the kidneys are responsible for the majority of drug clearance from the body, the reduced function will slow drug clearance rates.

Immune system: As a person ages, there is a definite shift in immune system capabilities. Older adults lose resistance to the development of infection and will demonstrate different signs and symptoms. The number of circulatory white blood cells diminishes, leaving fewer white cells to fight off invading organisms. The remaining white blood cells will slow down in their response time to ingest an organism. Finally, the release of endotoxins from white blood cells into the plasma will be delayed, which is actually the cause of a fever.

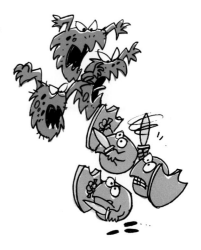

Other Special Needs for Older Adults

If truly successful IV therapy is to be provided, other age-related changes should be considered beyond the identified age-physiologic changes in the major body systems. These considerations relate to sensory and central nervous system changes. An older person's cooperation with procedures may be greatly improved when the health care provider practices a few simple steps. When a person's hearing, vision, mental processing ability, or emotional state changes, information received by the person is often distorted, incomplete, or confusing. This misunderstood information will create a reaction or patient response that is one of resistance, fear, agitation, combativeness, or any combination.

What You DO

Venipuncture Preparation

Knock on the patient's room door before entry, and call the patient by name. Lightly touch the patient's arm to ensure that the patient knows that **you** are in the room. Speak slowly and clearly at a moderate level once the patient's attention is gained. Talking louder only makes the words more difficult for a person who is hard of hearing to understand. Face the patient so that he or she can see **your** lips, which is important if the patient cannot hear well. Explain **your** identity and the procedure to be performed, and gain the patient's permission. Give the older patient a few extra seconds to process and respond to information. The normal physiologic aging process creates a slowing down of a person's actions, thoughts, and emotions.

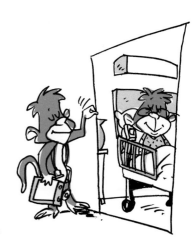

Practice proper aseptic technique, including proper hand washing, IV and site preparation, and central line care to prevent increasing the risk of infection. When cleaning with alcohol, avoid excessive rubbing and wetting of the skin. Alcohol is extremely drying and, when combined with the increased loss of natural moisture in the skin, leads to dryness and cracking.

Apply a tourniquet loosely over clothing to prevent overextension of the veins and to protect the skin from tearing or bruising. The prominent, large, and firm vein in an elderly person is not a good choice for venipuncture. This vein wall resists entry and, even if entered, may not allow for proper infusion because of the hardened (sclerosed) condition. These veins may be difficult to stabilize and will move away from a needle tip (rolling) during insertion. Identify medium to small veins that depress easily under the fingertips and refill quickly. This action will indicate a softer more resilient vein wall and improve the success of IV catheter placement. The veins in the mid-inner forearm area may be more accessible in older adults. The selection of a peripheral IV catheter with wings on the hub will improve device stabilization. Use a small 22- or 24-gauge catheter with a short length.

Because of the loss of tissue surrounding the vein, good vein stabilization must be done to prevent the vein from rolling. It is best to lower the angle on the IV device to approximately 5 to 10 degrees. This action will accommodate the loss of subcutaneous tissue and less on skin resistance.

Insertion Tips

Slow the speed and **apply less force** to enter the skin with the IV catheter. This technique minimizes the potential for perforating the back wall of the vein. Accessing a hand vein will require a slight increase in pressure to enter the vein with an IV catheter. **Avoid excess manipulation** of the catheter or "digging" for the vein. This caution is especially important in the mid-inner forearm area, resulting from the presence of nerves, tendons, and other structures that can be damaged. **Maintain vein traction** during entry into the skin and vein wall until a flashback is seen in the catheter flashback chamber. Decreased pulse pressure and slowed venous perfusion may result in minimal flashback during venipuncture. Maintain the traction until the catheter has been completely advanced into the vein. Release the tourniquet. With fragile veins, release the tourniquet after the flashback has been achieved to prevent hematoma formation at the insertion site. If the skin tension is released before the catheter is threaded, the rebound of the skin and vein being released may cause the catheter to rupture the vein. Avoid the catheter hub pushing against the insertion site; the pressure may tear the insertion site. Adding an extension to the catheter can reduce catheter movement and potential insertion site damage. Apply a skin protectant and allow to dry. Pad all connections with gauze. Because of the reduced elasticity of an older adult's skin, the amount of tape used to secure the IV catheter should be minimal. If tape is required, use hypoallergenic or paper tape. Transparent dressings work well and may require little additional tape.

Insertion Site Protection

The most challenging task is protecting an IV site or preventing catheters from being dislodged or pulled out. An approach of using more tape or "wrapping" a site is often performed to protect or maintain the peripheral IV. Wrapping an IV site with a gauze roll of any type is strongly discouraged and is against national standards for IV practice. This approach obscures the insertion site, may hide complication occurrence, and can cause injury. Future IV access may then be difficult, if not impossible.

If available in an institution, IV site protection is best done using a flexible mesh material, similar to the way in which burn dressings are secured. This netting comes in tube form and is available in different sizes. The mesh can be pulled over the insertion site and tubing while allowing good insertion site and extremity visibility. This material may also easily be removed for site inspection, is not restrictive, and will allow for full range of motion of the patient's hand or arm. A long-sleeve gown, sweater, or mitten could "hide" the site and help protect it. However, remember to always inspect the IV site at least hourly.

Care and Maintenance

Dressings that are not changed at appropriate intervals or are loose or "falling off" will expose the peripheral or central IV entry site to potentially life-threatening organisms.

It is essential to know the initial signs and symptoms that an elderly person will demonstrate when an infection is present. Because of the physiologic changes in the white blood cell numbers and function, a fever will **not** be the first sign of infection. A fever will not generally occur until day three of an infection, and most elderly patients who are diagnosed at this point are in septic shock and may die.

The first symptoms of infection are usually lethargy, slight confusion or disorientation (or both), and loss of appetite. Noting these occurrences early will help diagnose an infection and prevent the occurrence of sepsis and possible death. Be alert for any behavior shifts or changes in the patient that may indicate an infection. Any lack of appetite, reduced food intake, and excessive tiredness or sleeping will be other warning signs for which to be alerted. In combination, these three symptoms are often called the "classic picture of infection" in older adults.

Be on the alert for toxic signs from drugs given to older adults via IVs. Drugs delivered into the bloodstream will possibly exceed the proper levels if doses are not altered to fit the geriatric needs. Usually, drug doses are

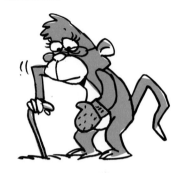

Using excess tape to secure an IV should be avoided in older adults because of the risk of skin and tissue damage when removed.

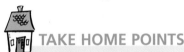

TAKE HOME POINTS

If restraint-type mittens are used, be sure to adhere to all policies for using patient restraints.

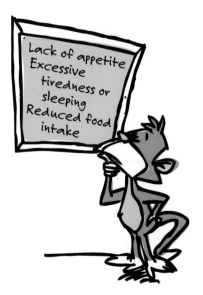

Lack of appetite
Excessive tiredness or sleeping
Reduced food intake

slightly reduced to avoid this toxic result. Monitor the elderly patient for unusual side effects such as the occurrence of confusion. This sign may indicate that the drug dose may need to be reduced.

To avoid the occurrence of circulatory overload, the rates of rehydration or IV fluid administration (for a person over the age of 65) should be ideally no more than 80 to 100 cc/hr. When medically appropriate and in the absence of cardiac or renal impairment, fluid rates over 100 cc/hr are prescribed. When this high volume occurs, the older person will need to be closely observed to prevent exceeding the body's ability to filter fluids through the kidneys.

The prolonged clearance of drugs from the body will increase the risk of toxicity if drug doses and administration time frames are not adjusted. Normal drug dosing times are often lengthened (e.g., an 8-hour dosing is delayed to a 10- or 12-hour dosing approach) to account for the prolonged clearing time. The elderly patient will still need to be monitored for signs and symptoms of drug toxicity.

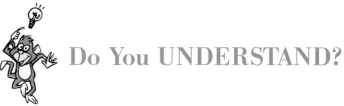

Do You UNDERSTAND?

DIRECTIONS: **Fill in the blanks with the correct arrow.**

    a. ↑
    b. ↓

1. The geriatric population is _____ and will continue to do so over the next 15 to 20 years.
2. A lack of awareness of the predictable physiologic system changes in older adults will _____ the risk for complications and adverse effects of IV delivery.
3. The work of the immune system _____ with age.
4. There is a _____ in collagen and subcutaneous fat in the skin of older adults.

DIRECTIONS: **Identify the following statements as** *true* **(T) or** *false* **(F) regarding changes in older adults that can affect IV therapy.**

5. _____ The vein is more elastic.

6. _____ Small veins and capillaries become thinner and more fragile.

7. _____ The liver reduces in size with aging.

8. _____ There is an increase in the filtration rate of the kidneys.

DIRECTIONS: **Match the statement in Column A with the rationale in Column B.**

Column A

9. _____ Apply a tourniquet loosely over clothing.

10. _____ Lower the angle on the IV device to 5 to 10 degrees.

11. _____ Use a flexible mesh dressing for IV site protection.

12. _____ Avoid using excessive tape at the IV site.

Column B

a. To avoid skin and tissue damage on removal

b. To accommodate for loss of subcutaneous tissue

c. To increase ease of site inspection

d. To protect skin from bruising or tearing

DIRECTIONS: **Provide the answer to the following question.**

13. What are the early symptoms of infection in the older adult? (*Circle each symptom from the following list.*)

Fever

Cachexia

Coma

Elevated serum creatinine level

Hypertension

Loss of appetite

Lethargy

Rash on body

Slight confusion

DIRECTIONS: **Find and circle these words in the following puzzle.**

central nervous	liver	sensory
fragile skin	mental processing	thicker vein
hearing	reduced filtration	vision
less resistant		

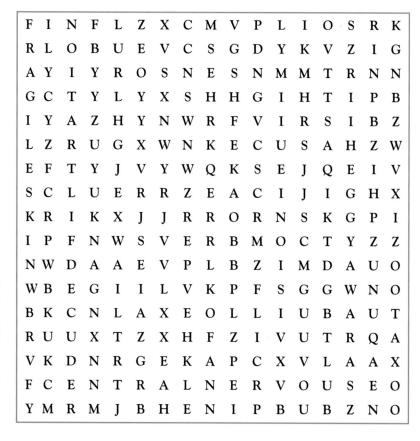

F I N F L Z X C M V P L I O S R K
R L O B U E V C S G D Y K V Z I G
A Y I Y R O S N E S N M M T R N N
G C T Y L X S H H G I H T I P B
I Y A Z H Y N W R F V I R S I B Z
L Z R U G X W N K E C U S A H Z W
E F T Y J V Y W Q K S E J Q E I V
S C L U E R R Z E A C I J I G H X
K R I K X J J R R O R N S K G P I
I P F N W S V E R B M O C T Y Z Z
N W D A A E V P L B Z I M D A U O
W B E G I I L V K P F S G G W N O
B K C N L A X E O L L I U B A U T
R U U X T Z X H F Z I V U T R Q A
V K D N R G E K A P C X V L A A X
F C E N T R A L N E R V O U S E O
Y M R M J B H E N I P B U B Z N O

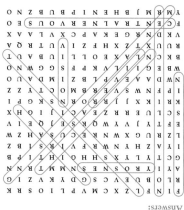

Answers:

8 Community-Based Infusion Therapy

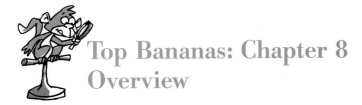

Top Bananas: Chapter 8 Overview

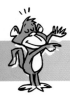

What IS Community-Based Infusion Therapy?

Community-based infusion therapy is therapy that is implemented, by routes that can be safely and cost-effectively provided, within the home environment. These therapies are implemented through intravenous (IV), subcutaneous, intrathecal, and gastric routes and provide products that include, but are not limited to, antibiotics, chemotherapy, blood products, substances for nutritional support, and medications for pain management. Safety for the patient and his or her family is of primary concern when considering this type of therapy as a treatment option.

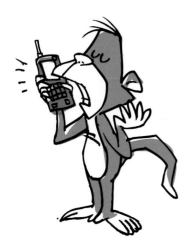

 What You NEED TO KNOW

An evaluation of several key components is necessary to identify if the patient is a candidate for care that is to be provided in the home. Of these, the two most important components are the home environment and the patient or caregivers.

Evaluating the Safety of the Home Environment

Several factors have to be evaluated in the home. It is necessary to evaluate the following areas to confirm that therapy can be provided safely in the home environment.

- Is there a telephone in the home? The patient must have access to a telephone for several reasons. Most importantly, the patient must have access to 911 service in case of an emergency. Is 911 service available in the patient's home area? Is the patient close to a facility that can provide the emergency care that may be needed? Additionally, the patient needs two-way communication with the service provider. The service provider must be available 24 hours a day in case the patient has a problem or a question. Many problems can be handled over the telephone; but if not, the provider must have someone who is available to go to the home to resolve the problem. The service provider must be able to get in touch with the patient to set up appointments, provide follow-up care, get the inventory of supplies in the home, and arrange for nurse visits and deliveries.

- Does the home have electricity? Electricity is necessary for several reasons. First, it is important that there be adequate lighting for the patient or caregiver to be able to perform the necessary procedures that are involved. Second, refrigeration of medications or other products is needed in most circumstances.

- Is there running water—both hot and cold? The caregiver, whether he or she is the patient, a family member, or friend, will need to practice good hand-washing techniques before assembling syringes, infusion products, and initiating the infusion.

TAKE HOME POINTS

Many of the infusion products must be refrigerated until they are warmed to room temperature before being infused. Additionally, products remain stable for a longer period when refrigerated. Electricity is necessary for most infusion pumps to operate for long periods of time. Some infusion pumps can operate on battery power but require an electrical outlet to be charged adequately.

TAKE HOME POINTS

If running water is not available, then use alcohol-based hand rub as directed by agency policy to prevent infection.

Caregiver Criteria

The caregiver must meet certain criteria, whether he or she is the patient, a friend, or family member. The caregiver must:

1. Be motivated.
2. Be willing to participate in patient care.
3. Be willing to perform functions required for patient care.
4. Have the cognitive ability to perform required procedures.
5. Be able to solve problems independently.
6. Be able to discern when to call for help.
7. Have the manual dexterity to manipulate equipment (e.g., syringes, tubing, pumps).
8. Have adequate visual acuity to perform procedures.
9. Have adequate hand-eye coordination.

Nursing Responsibilities

The professional nurse needs to know that entering a patient's home for infusion therapy is quite different from the clean or sterile clinical settings to which the nurse is accustomed. Some homes may not be clean and may have insects and other pests. It is important that the nurse accept the patient in the home setting nonjudgmentally, while planning the changes that will be necessary to render adequate treatment. For example, the nurse may have to make changes in the environment to start the infusion, such as securing privacy and obtaining proper lighting. The obstacles to treating the patient in the home must be overcome before treatment can begin. It is important that the nurse make these changes gently and with a positive attitude so that the patient will not be offended.

The nurse is also responsible for assessing the home for hazards that can be eliminated for the safety of the patient and family. The nurse must realize that this precaution is taken in the spirit of advocacy for the sake of the patient and not feel "nosey" when inspecting the home for hazards. When necessary, the nurse should secure help from social services and other church and community agencies to provide a safe environment for the patient. For example, the nurse may note that there are no handrails on the front or back steps to assist a frail patient in walking in or out of the house. Most communities have volunteers who are willing to help people in need when requested by the provider. The nurse must do whatever is necessary to provide a conducive environment for home infusion therapy and overall safety of the patient. The nurse must always endeavor to gain the trust and confidence of the patient and caregiver.

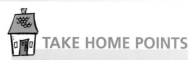

TAKE HOME POINTS

People with arthritis may have difficulty performing some of the necessary duties.

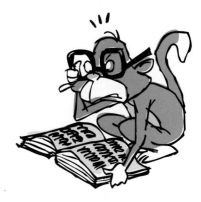

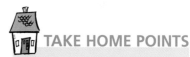

TAKE HOME POINTS

Possible home hazards include roaming animals who can disrupt a sterile field and overloaded circuits into which too many devices are plugged.

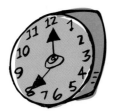

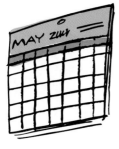

When teaching the patient and caregiver about possible complications of infusion therapy, it is important that the patient and caregiver understand that the provider is available 24 hours a day and 7 days a week and should be called immediately if any signs and symptoms of complications occur. Some patients may tend to wait to see if symptoms subside or delay calling because they do not want to "bother" the nurse who is on call. It is essential that the patient and caregiver understand that early notification and intervention are keys to success and may prevent serious problems. It is necessary for the nurse to communicate the importance of prompt notification so that any problems that occur may be kept to a minimum. Although it is important to teach about signs and symptoms of complications (see "What You DO" later in this chapter), it is also necessary to teach in a manner that will not frighten the patient and caregiver to the point at which they cannot function properly.

What You DO

Patient and Caregiver Education

The home care nurse must teach the patient and caregiver at least five basic principles of care. The **first basic principle** that needs to be explained and demonstrated to the person performing the infusion procedure deals with what is "sterile" and what is "clean."

- Items that are sterile can be handled only with sterile gloves. If an item becomes contaminated—**simply do not use it.** Throw it away. Specific items that need to be identified as sterile include needles, syringe hubs, tubing spikes, the end of tubings, and contents of sterile kits. Additionally, some needleless systems have certain areas that are sterile. For example, some systems use a cap to cover a port that is used for flushing. When the cap is removed, the port is sterile. Use a new sterile cap to cover the port after use.
- Other items are considered clean. These items can be handled with clean, washed hands without the danger of contaminating the infusion. Examples of clean items include tubings, syringe barrels, the caps covering needles, infusion devices, and pumps.

The nurse sometimes requires a language translator to assist in teaching. Suggestions for resources include neighbors, local hospital, local church, local chamber of commerce, the Internet, and AT&T phone company.

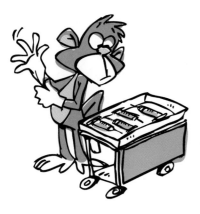

The **second basic principle** is this: "If you are going to stick a needle into it, clean it with alcohol first." Some infusions may require additives. For example, multivitamins may need to be added to parenteral nutrition by being drawn up in a syringe using a needle. Before puncturing the container cap with a needle, wipe the cap with alcohol. Similarly, before the needle is inserted into the additive port on the container, the port must be wiped with alcohol. Prepare skin appropriately (see Chapter 2).

Some needleless systems use a valve system that is not covered with a cap. With this type of system, the valve should be wiped with alcohol before it is accessed with a syringe.

The **third basic principle** is that the person providing the care must receive a full demonstration of what is expected to be done. This demonstration should include verbal instructions that explain the procedure, identification of sterile items, and the reasons that things need to be done in a certain way. Basic principles must be followed to ensure that the safety and well being of the patient is not jeopardized. For example, inserting a contaminated tubing spike into a bag of sterile fluid might potentially lead to a state of sepsis for the patient.

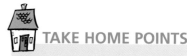

TAKE HOME POINTS

People learn in different ways. Some people will learn best with written instructions, some with pictures and drawings, and others will learn from watching and observing.

Instructions for the caregiver should include a written list of the items necessary for the care to be provided, as well as step-by-step instructions for the care.

The **fourth basic principle** is that the person performing the infusion must give a return demonstration of the entire infusion procedure. The caregiver needs to be able to verbalize the steps in the procedure and demonstrate a basic understanding of the rationale for the order in which the steps are performed. When possible, use teaching tools for the patient and caregiver that include illustrations or pictures of the procedure to be done. This approach provides strong reinforcement of the teaching after the nurse is gone. Written directions for maintaining and operating the infusion must be provided in a manner that the patient and caregiver find understandable. The directions or instructions should be posted in an easily accessible location, such as at the patient's bedside or on the refrigerator door.

The **fifth basic principle** is that the patient or caregiver needs to be instructed on potential problems. The care provider must teach basic troubleshooting skills and problem solving techniques. Teach the caregiver who, when, and how to call for help.

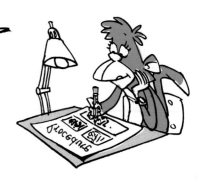

Prepare written instructions in 14-point type or larger for older adults.

The provider should be notified if any of the following signs and symptoms occurs:

- Pain or swelling at the infusion site
- Changes in respiratory or heart rates
- Shortness of breath
- Dizziness
- Headache
- Facial flushing

- Loss of consciousness
- Chills
- Fever
- Nausea and vomiting
- Anxiety

The nurse must always prominently display the provider's phone number so the patient has easy access to it 24 hours a day.

Community-based infusion therapy is always user and therapy specific.

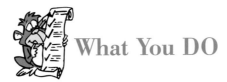

What You DO

Nursing Care

All of the information that applies to IV therapy also applies to home infusion therapy. However, there are a few additional nuances of which the home care nurse needs to be aware.

The nurse receiving the prescription for home infusion therapy must first call and make an appointment with the patient or caregiver in the home. Timing is critical when the patient is being discharged from the hospital with prescriptions to continue therapy. Timing is also critical when the patient is in pain and awaiting the initiation of infusion for pain control. The nurse must be sensitive to these important aspects of patient care and respond quickly and efficiently when receiving prescriptions for infusion in the home setting.

The nurse must obtain the solutions to be infused and additives from the pharmacy that is contracted to supply the medications. The nurse must also coordinate delivery of all supplies and equipment to ensure timely delivery so that treatment can begin promptly.

When arriving at the patient's home, the nurse should arrange for patient privacy, away from the main traffic pattern in the home. Frequently, the nurse will move the patient to the bedroom to set up a work space. If the caregiver will be present, the private location must be large enough for three people plus the supplies and workspace.

TAKE HOME POINTS

Infusions to control pain require assessment for severity of pain on a 1 to 10 scale, as well as respiratory rate and pattern.

TAKE HOME POINTS

If Narcan is prescribed, it should be given slowly IV and stopped once the respiratory rate reaches equal or greater than seven breaths per minute or to the level the institution's policy indicates.

The nurse must next obtain adequate lighting for the task. This provision may mean that lamps may need to be brought in from other rooms in the house to illuminate the workspace.

The nurse must secure adequate workspace. Do not be shy about moving the patient's personal belongings as needed to create an uncluttered, safe workspace. Be sure to place the patient's things back in their original order when the task is complete.

While making these changes in the environment, the nurse should be careful to explain the need for ample work area and adequate lighting to the patient or caregiver.

Next, the nurse must ask that all pets in the home be secured in a separate room or kennel so that the work area does not become contaminated with pet hair or by a pet actually leaping onto the work area itself. Take extra time to make sure that all pets are restrained before risking the loss of a sterile field to a playful kitten!

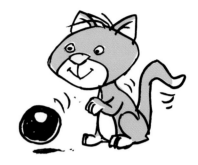

It is recommended that windows and doors be closed and that fans be turned off during the procedures to lessen the likelihood of contamination from flying particles, including pet hair.

Before beginning, the nurse must follow the provider's hand-washing policy. Hand-washing time provides an opportunity to teach good hand-washing techniques to the patient or caregiver. The nurse should use the liquid soap and paper towels provided by the agency that are carried in the home-visit supply bag. The patient or caregiver should use the soap available in the home. If paper towels are not available, they should use a clean cloth for drying.

During the time while the nurse is present for the infusion procedure, the patient should be asked to avoid all disturbances. For instance, if the phone rings, let the answering machine pick up a message, or just let the phone ring. The patient will not be able to answer the phone, pager, or doorbell while a procedure is being performed. It is helpful for the patient to make frequent callers aware of the need for an uninterrupted time while the nurse is present.

These measures are put in place to maximize the patient's safety and well being and to avoid complications in treatment.

A container for disposal of sharps is provided by the agency. If a container is not available, the nurse may use empty, hard plastic containers, such as the bottle in which liquid laundry detergent comes. The container should be disposed according to agency procedure based on local, state, and federal requirements.

⚠ Extravasation and anaphylaxis are two of the most serious problems that can occur in community-based infusion therapy.

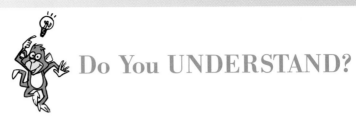

Do You UNDERSTAND?

DIRECTIONS: **Unscramble the following words to find the essential factors that must exist for successful infusion therapy in the home.**

1. _____ (ratwe)
2. _____ (openhteel)
3. _____ (tycileectir)
4. _____ (vegaicerr)
5. _____ _____ (lasuvi ticauy)

DIRECTIONS: **Fill in the blanks to complete the statement.**

The five basic principles of care for community-based infusion therapy are:

6. Teach the patient and caregiver which items are _____ and which items are _____, including the differences in handling the items.

7. If the nurse is going to stick a needle into it, _____ it with _____ first.

8. The person providing the care must receive a full _____ of the care that is to be given.

9. The person performing the infusion must give a _____ _____ of the entire process.

10. The patient and caregiver need to be instructed on _____ _____ _____.

DIRECTIONS: **Identify the following statements as *true* (T) or *false* (F).**

11. _____ Timing is critical when beginning IV therapy in the home.

12. _____ The secretary for the provider is the best person to coordinate items needed for the home infusion.

13. _____ Hand washing and proper disposal of waste are two important aspects of care in the home.

14. _____ The nurse must first survey the home setting to find an appropriate space to set up to begin the infusion.

15. _____ Good lighting in the home is not necessary because starting an IV is a routine task for the home infusion nurse.

16. _____ The nurse should allow the patient to hold a pet during the IV starting procedure to keep the patient calm.

17. _____ Pain is often managed in the home through proper infusion therapy.

18. _____ It is important to teach the patient and caregiver proper disposal of sharps.

19. _____ If the patient experiences pain and swelling at the infusion site, it is acceptable to wait until the next nurse's visit to report the problem.

20. _____ The nurse should leave a phone number for the patient and caregiver to call for assistance 24 hours per day and 7 days a week.

Appendix

Locations of Intravenous Product Manufacturers

PRODUCTS	MANUFACTURERS	LOCATIONS
IV House Dome and Ultra Dressing	IV House	St. Louis, MO
StatLock	Venetec International	San Diego, CA
PasV™	Boston Scientific Corporation	Natick, MA
Hickman®, Hohn®, Leonard®, Broviac®, Groshong®	Bard	Salt Lake City, UT
Persist, Insyte, Angiocath	Becton, Dickinson and Company	Franklin Lakes, NJ
Steri Strip, Tegaderm	3M	St. Paul, MN
ELA-max	Ferndale Laboratories	Ferndale, MI
EMLA	AstraZeneca PLC	Wilmington, DE
ChloraPrep	Medi-Flex	Overland Park, KS
IV Prep	Smith & Nephew	Largo, FL

References

Chapter 1: Equipment and Infusion Regulation Devices

Booker MF, Ignatavicius DD: *Infusion therapy techniques & medications*, Philadelphia, 1996, WB Saunders.

Hankins J et al: *Infusion therapy in clinical practice*, ed 2, Philadelphia, 2001, WB Saunders.

Infusion Nursing Society: Infusion nursing standards of practice, *J Intraven Nurs* 23(6S):S1, 2000.

Macklin DC: What's physics got to do with it? A review of the physical principles of fluid administration, *J Vascul Access Devices* 4(2):7, 1999.

O'Grady NP et al: Draft guideline for the prevention of intravascular catheter-related infections, *Am J Infect Control* 30(8):476, 2002.

Trissel LA: *Handbook on injectable drugs*, ed 11, Bethesda, 2000, American Society of Health-System Pharmacists.

Chapter 2: Principles of Peripheral Venous Therapy

Brown J, Larson M: Pain during insertion of peripheral intravenous catheters with and without intradermal lidocaine, *Clin Nurse Spec* 13(6):283, 1999.

Catney MR et al: Relationship between peripheral intravenous catheter dwell time and the development of phlebitis and infiltration, *J Infus Nurs* 24(5):332, 2001.

Chernecky C, Macklin D, Murphy-Ende K: *Real-world nursing survival guide: fluids & electrolytes*, Philadelphia, 2002, WB Saunders.

Fetzer S: Reducing the pain of venipuncture, *J Perianesth Nurs* 14(2):95, 1999.

Hankins J et al: *Infusion therapy in clinical practice*, ed 2, Philadelphia, 2001, WB Saunders.

Infusion Nursing Society: Infusion nursing standards of practice, *J Intraven Nurs* 23(6S):S1, 2000.

LeBlanc A, Cobbett S: Traditional practice versus evidence-based practice for IV skin preparation, *Can J Infect Control* 15(1):9, 2000.

Macklin DC: *Basic IV therapy*, www.ceuzone.com, 2001.

Macklin DC: What's physics got to do with it? A review of the physical principles of fluid administration, *J Vascul Access Devices* 4(2):7, 1999.

O'Grady NP et al: Draft guideline for the prevention of intravascular catheter-related infections, *Am J Infect Control* 30(8):476, 2002.

Vengelen-Tyler V: *Technical manual*, ed 12, Bethesda, 1996, American Association of Blood Banks.

Witmer DR: Promoting rational drug use through the ASHP commission on therapeutics, *Am J Hosp Pharm* 51(12):1536, 1994.

Chapter 3: Peripheral Complications

Berghammer P et al: Doxetaxel extravasation, *Support Care Cancer* 9(2):131, 2001.

Fabian B: Intravenous complication: infiltration, *J Intraven Nurs* 23(4):229, 2000.

Hanchett M: Infusion outcome analysis in the new millennium: what advanced practitioners need to know, *J Vascul Access Devices* 6(1):18, 2001.

Hankins J et al: *Infusion therapy in clinical practice*, ed 2, Philadelphia, 2001, WB Saunders.

Infusion Nursing Society: Infusion nursing standards of practice, *J Intraven Nurs* 23(6S):S1, 2000.

Lawson T: Vein trauma during catheter advancement and its possible consequences to the condition of the patient, *J Vascul Access Devices* 3(1):22, 1998.

Macklin DC: Phlebitis, *Am J Nurs* 103(2):55, 2003.

Maki DG, Mermel LA: Infections due to infusion therapy. In Bennett JV, Brachman PS, editors: *Hospital infections*, ed 4, Philadelphia, 1998, Lippincott.

Smith JP: Thrombotic complications in intravenous access, *J Intraven Nurs* 21(2):96, 1998.

Whang SW, Lee SH: Intralesional steroids reduce inflammation from extravasated chemotherapeutic agents, *Br J Dermatol* 145(4):680, 2001.

Yucha CB et al: Characterization of intravenous infiltrates, *Appl Nurs Res* 4(4):184, 1991.

Yucha CB, Hastings-Tolsma M, Szeverenyi NM: Effect of elevation on intravenous extravasations, *J Intraven Nurs* 17(5):231, 1994.

Chapter 4: Principles of Central Venous Therapy

Baranowski L: Central venous access devices: current technologies, uses and management strategies, *J Intraven Nurs* 16(3):167, 1993.

Chernecky C: Satisfaction versus dissatisfaction with venous access devices in outpatient oncology: a pilot study, *Oncol Nurs Forum* 28(10):1613, 2001.

Chernecky C, Macklin D, Nugent K, Waller J et al: Preferences in choosing venous access devices by intravenous and oncology nurses, *J Vascul Access Devices* 8(4):35, 2003.

Chernecky C, Macklin D, Nugent K, Waller J et al: The need for shared decision-making in the selection of vascular access devices: an assessment of patients and clinicians, *J Vascul Access Devices* 7(3):34, 2002.

Gahart BL, Nazareno AR: *Intravenous medications*, ed 17, St Louis, 2001, Mosby.

Hankins J et al: *Infusion therapy in clinical practice*, ed 2, Philadelphia, 2001, WB Saunders.

Infusion Nursing Society: Infusion nursing standards of practice, *J Intraven Nurs* 23(6S):S1, 2000.

Kim DK, Gottesman MH, Forero A: The CVC removal distress syndrome. An unappreciated complication of central venous catheter removal, *Am Surg* 64(4):344, 1998.

Kluger DM, Maki DG: The relative risk of intravascular device related bloodstream infections in adults, *Abstracts of the 39th Interscience Conference on Antimicrobial Agents and Chemotherapy*, 514, 1999.

Macklin D: How to manage PICCs, *Am J Nurs* 97(9):26, 1997.

Macklin D: *Ports*, www.ceuzone.com, 2000.

Macklin D: Removing PICCs, *Am J Nurs* 100(1):52, 2000.

O'Grady NP et al: Draft guideline for the prevention of intravascular catheter-related infections, *Am J Infect Control* 30(8):476, 2002.

Vengelen-Tyler V, editor: *Technical manual*, ed 12, Bethesda, 1996, American Association of Blood Banks.

Chapter 5: Central Venous Catheter Complications

Collin GR: Decreasing catheter colonization through the use of an antiseptic-impregnated catheter. A continuous quality improvement project, *Chest* 115(6):1632, 1999.

Maki DG et al: Prevention of central venous catheter-related bloodstream infection by use of an antiseptic-impregnated catheter. A randomized, controlled trial, *Ann Int Med* 127(4):257, 1997.

Pai MP, Pendland SL, Danziger LH: Antimicrobial-coated/bonded and impregnated intravascular catheters, *Ann Pharmacother* 35(10):1255, 2001.

Pearson M: Guideline for prevention of intravascular device-related infections, *Am J Infect Control* 24(4):262, 1996.

Chapter 6: Pediatric Patient

Brennan A: Caring for children during procedures: a review of the literature, *Pediatr Nurs* 20(5):451, 1994.

Duck S: Neonatal intravenous therapy, *J Intraven Nurs* 20(3):121, 1997.

Critical care procedures. A guide to pediatric fluid replacement and maintenance, *Dimens Crit Care Nurs* 19(4):24, 2000.

Fanurik D, Koh JL, Schmitz ML: Distraction techniques combined with EMLA: effects of IV insertion pain and distress in children, *Child Health Care* 29(2):87, 2000.

Frederick V: Pediatric IV therapy: soothing the patient, *RN* 54(12):40, 1991.

Furdon SA: Operationalizing Donna Wong's principle of atraumatic care: pain management protocol in the NICU, *Pediatr Nurs* 24(4):336, 1998.

Hanrahan KS et al: Evaluation of saline for IV locks in children, *Pediatr Nurs* 20(6):549, 1994.

Hutchinson D: Pediatric IV therapy: starting the line, *RN* 54(12):43, 1991.

Infusion Nursing Society: Infusion nursing standards of practice, *J Intraven Nurs* 23(6S):S1, 2000.

O'Grady NP et al: Draft guideline for the prevention of intravascular catheter-related infections, *Am J Infect Control* 30(8):476, 2002.

Smith AB, Wilkinson-Faulk D: Factors affecting the life span of peripheral intravenous lines in hospitalized infants, *Pediatr Nurs* 20(6):543, 1994.

Chapter 7: Older Adult Patient

Coulter K: Intravenous therapy for the elderly patient: implications for the intravenous nurse, *J Intraven Nurs* 15:S18, 1992.

Gahart BL, Nazareno AR: *Intravenous medications*, ed 17, St Louis, 2001, Mosby.

Hand H: Continuing professional development: fluid management. The use of intravenous therapy, *Geriatr Nurs Home Care* 11(9):43, 2001.

Hankins J et al: *The infusion nurses society infusion therapy in clinical practice*, ed 2, Philadelphia, 2001, WB Saunders.

Infusion Nursing Society: Infusion nursing standards of practice, *J Intraven Nurs* 23(6S):S1, 2000.

Jones KC: Maintaining infusion therapy services in the long-term care setting, *J Infus Nurs* 24(6):381, 2001.

Matteson MA, McConnell ES: *Gerontological nursing concepts and practice*, ed 2, Philadelphia, 1996, WB Saunders.

Saxon SV, Etten MJ: *Physical change & aging: a guide for the helping professions*, ed 3, New York, 1994, Tiresias Press.

Weinstein SM: *Plumer's principles & practice of intravenous therapy*, ed 7, Philadelphia, 2001, Lippincott.

Whitehouse MJ: Nursing assessment of the elderly patient, *J Intraven Nurs* 15:S14, 1992.

Whitehouse MJ: The physiology of aging, *J Intraven Nurs* 15:S7, 1992.

Chapter 8: Community-Based Infusion Therapy

Kayley J: Clinical update. Home IV antibiotic therapy, *Geriatr Nurs Home Care* 10(6):25, 2000.

Macduff C, Leslie A, West B: Ambulatory chemotherapy—toward best community practice, *J Community Nurs* 15(7):24, 2001.

Marvin P, Acevedo M: Regional excellence in intravenous therapy: it all began with community intravenous therapy education, *J Intraven Nurs* 14(2):123, 1991.

O'Halloran L: The development of a theory and evidence-based home infusion program, *Canadian Intravenous Nurses Association 26th Annual Conference: Official Journal of the Canadian Intravenous Nurses Association*, 1716, 2001.

Sexton JS, Seldomridge L: The characteristics and clinical practices of nurses who perform home infusion therapies, *J Infus Nurs* 25(3):176, 2002.

Illustration Credits

Pages 5, 6, 10: Redrawn from Booker MF, Ignatavicius DD: *Infusion therapy techniques & medications,* Philadelphia, 1996, WB Saunders.

Pages 7, 32, 33, 34, 35, 36, 45, 49, 50, 51, 53, 131, 134: Redrawn from Macklin D: PICC care & maintenance, www.ceuzone.com, Professional Learning Systems, Inc., 2002.

Pages 32, 33, 34, 35, 36, 45, 49, 50, 51, 53, 170: Redrawn from Macklin D: Basic IV therapy, www.ceuzone.com, Professional Learning Systems, Inc., 2002.

Pages 84, 99, 109: Redrawn from Macklin D: Implanted ports, www.ceuzone.com, Professional Learning Systems, Inc., 2002.

Pages 86, 95, 97, 164, 165: Courtesy of Bard Access Systems, Salt Lake City, Utah.

Pages 87, 97: Courtesy Boston Scientific Corporation, Natick, Massachusetts.

Pages 126, 134: Courtesy Nancy Moureau, PICC Excellence, Inc., Orange Park, Florida.

Pages 135, 136: Redrawn from Herbst SL, Kaplan LK, McKinnon BT: Infusion, 4:S1-S32, 1998.

Page 162: Courtesy of Gail Egan Sansivero, MS, ANP, AOCN. The Institute for Vascular Health and Disease, Albany Medical Center, Albany, New York.

Page 188: Courtesy of IV House, St. Louis, Missouri.

NCLEX Section

CHAPTER *1* Equipment and Infusion Regulation
          Devices

1. Which of the following is an advantage of a glass solution container and not a plastic solution container?
   1 Light weight
   2 Easy to store
   3 Does not allow medications to degrade the container
   4 Is not breakable

2. Which of the following medications should be placed in a glass solution container when being administered via IV to a patient?
   1 D_5W
   2 Regular insulin
   3 Cimetidine (Tagamet)
   4 Gentamycin

3. Which of the following containers does **not** require the use of a vented administration set?
   1 Plastic
   2 Semirigid
   3 Glass
   4 Stainless steel

4. The nurse has opened the outer wrap of a 1000-ml plastic container of $D_5^1/2NS$. Pooling of fluid is noted inside the wrapper. What should be done?
   1 Hang this bag of fluid.
   2 Hang this bag of fluid, but decrease the prescribed rate by 20%.
   3 Return the bag to central supply for credit and hang another bag of $D_5^1/2NS$.
   4 Remove 50% of the fluid from the bag and give the other 50% at the prescribed rate.

5. When hanging a primary solution, it should be elevated to:
   1 Even with the patient's heart
   2 12 inches above the patient's heart
   3 36 inches above the patient's heart
   4 24 inches above the patient's heart

6. Which of the following items are included in all administration sets?
   1 Tubing, drip chamber, add-ons, filter, and end syringe
   2 Clamp, spike, drop orifice, and membrane filter
   3 Drop orifice, clamp, tubing, injection port, and stopcock
   4 Spike, drop orifice, drip chamber, tubing, and clamp

7. Which of the following items in an administration set is used to calculate infusion rates and is located at the top of the drip chamber?
   1 Spike
   2 Drop orifice
   3 Secondary set
   4 Clamp

8. What is the correct number of drops per minute for an infusing D_5NS at 120 cc per hour with a drop factor of 10 drops per milliliter?
   1 10 drops per minute
   2 20 drops per minute
   3 60 drops per minute
   4 120 drops per minute

9. The name for the connection at the end of an IV tubing that screws onto the IV catheter is called a:
   1 Slip connector
   2 Clamp
   3 Back-check valve
   4 Leur lock

219

10. Which of the following is not a type of filter?
    1 Membrane
    2 Screen
    3 Depth
    4 Stopcock

11. What type of add-on equipment is added to an IV catheter to permit the infusion of two or three infusions and is known as *multi-flow* or **Y** designs?
    1 Extension sets
    2 Depth filters
    3 Connectors
    4 Membrane filters

12. In what system of infusion regulation is the pressure gradient generated by the height of the IV bag?
    1 Mechanical system
    2 Electronic system
    3 Gravity system
    4 Elastometric pump system

13. Which of the following systems used to generate flow rate has the advantage of free-flow prevention?
    1 Mechanical
    2 Electronic
    3 Elastometric
    4 Gravity

14. Mr. Jacobs has a peripheral IV placed near his right wrist. He begins typing on his computer, and 3 minutes later, while he is still typing on his computer, an alarm goes off on his electronic IV pump. The alarm is most likely signaling:
    1 Low battery
    2 Air in the line
    3 Door ajar
    4 Occlusion

15. Mrs. Kuo has a primary IV with a roller clamp. The nurse notices that her fluid rate is decreasing. What is the first nursing intervention?
    1 Restart the IV.
    2 Move and readjust the roller clamp.
    3 Add a resistor to the IV line.
    4 Lower the height of the IV bag.

CHAPTER *2:* Principles of Peripheral Venous Therapy

1. To determine the vein location for peripheral IV insertion, which of the following does **not** need to be assessed?
    1 Mental status
    2 Patient diagnosis
    3 Chest x-ray
    4 Type of therapy

2. Mrs. Hernandez is scheduled to receive 4 months of IV chemotherapy for cervical cancer. This length of therapy is defined as:
    1 Short-term
    2 Intermediate
    3 Long-term
    4 Futuristic

3. A person with diabetes mellitus is at risk for problems with obtaining peripheral venous access because hyperglycemia activates plasma proteins that cause:
    1 Vasoconstriction
    2 Vasodilation
    3 Heart failure
    4 Chemical phlebitis

4. A person who is allergic to latex should avoid which of the following foods?
    1 Beef jerky
    2 Lettuce
    3 Bananas
    4 Ice cream

5. Mr. Holliman is not currently being prescribed or taking any medications. However, he is about to begin receiving two different types of IV antibiotics for an infection of a newly inserted tricuspid heart valve. What laboratory results should be assessed before beginning the antibiotic treatment?
    1 Serum calcium
    2 Serum potassium
    3 C & S
    4 Prothrombin time

6. Which medication places a patient at high risk for hematoma formation after venipuncture?
   1 Acetaminophen (Tylenol)
   2 Gentamicin (Garamycin)
   3 Digoxin (Lanoxin)
   4 Acetylsalicylic acid (aspirin)

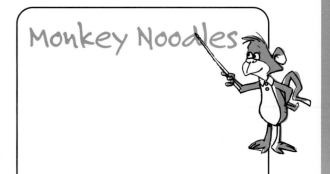

7. The nurse is scheduled to withdraw five tubes of blood peripherally from a patient who is highly allergic to latex. What equipment (necessary to perform this peripheral venipuncture) should the nurse ensure is not made from latex?
   1 Disposable syringe
   2 Injection port of blood tube
   3 Tourniquet
   4 2 × 2 gauze

8. A patient has just been admitted to the emergency room after spending 3 days lost in the hot desert of Arizona, and he is unconscious. What information does the nurse have that would remind him or her that venous distention will be difficult?
   1 The patient cannot speak.
   2 The patient is dehydrated.
   3 Men have less venous distention, in general, than women.
   4 Arizona is at a high altitude, and veins tend to collapse under altitude pressure.

9. Mrs. Sanderson is scheduled to have a right mastectomy tomorrow for stage 3 breast cancer. She is right-handed, and the nurse is to start her IV preoperatively. In which appendage should he or she start the peripheral IV?
   1 Left arm
   2 Right arm
   3 Left foot
   4 Right foot

10. Mr. Champion has been admitted with a right-sided brain stroke and left-sided paralysis. He is hyponatremic and requires a peripheral IV started immediately. In which arm should the IV be started?
    1 The left arm is the correct location.
    2 The right arm is the correct location.
    3 Do not start the IV; it is too risky.
    4 Call the physician and state that this patient needs an arterial line inserted.

CHAPTER *3:* Peripheral Complications

1. Which areas are important to assess in relation to the early detection of complications from a peripheral IV?
   1 Administration set-up, insertion site, dressing, and patient response
   2 Flow rate, insertion site, and type of health insurance
   3 Administration tubing, IV catheter, and chest x-ray results
   4 Fluid container, insertion site, and dressing

2. A patient is receiving a continuous heparin infusion. The electronic pump is continually beeping occlusion. The nurse should:
   1 Get another pump.
   2 Restart the IV.
   3 Take the heparin off the pump and infuse by gravity.
   4 Assess the administration set, dressing, and IV for possible constrictions.

3. The gravity low solution of D_5W is not infusing at the prescribed infusion rate. The nurse disconnects the IV line at the IV catheter site and notices that the D_5W flows freely. This situation indicates that the problem area is the:
   1 Administration set
   2 Patient's diastolic blood pressure
   3 IV catheter
   4 Type of IV solution (D_5W)

4. Which of the following is a potential cause of peripheral IV infiltration?
   1 Good dressing care
   2 Good vein elasticity
   3 Large size catheter in a small vein
   4 Low angle IV insertion technique

5. A patient has an infiltrated peripheral IV on her right lower dorsal forearm. Which anatomic location should **not** be accessed to restart another IV catheter?
   1 Left forearm
   2 Left hand area
   3 Right hand area
   4 Right ventral upper forearm

6. Electronic pumps do **not** recognize:
   1 That the infusion is complete
   2 In-line occlusion
   3 Air in the line
   4 Infiltration

7. With hypotonic or isotonic solutions, what type of compress is used on peripheral IV site infiltrations?
   1 Hot/dry
   2 Cold
   3 Hot/wet
   4 Applying compresses do not affect reabsorption time.

8. Which of the following is a potential vesicant?
   1 Dilantin
   2 Amphotericin B
   3 Furosemide (Lasix)
   4 Multivitamin solution

9. Which of the following 1000-ml dextrose solutions is considered a potential vesicant?
   1 D_5W
   2 $D_5\frac{1}{2}NS$
   3 20% dextrose
   4 D_5LR with 10 mEq potassium chloride

10. Which of the following symptoms indicates phlebitis?
    1 Cool skin, pain, and swelling
    2 Ecchymosis, edema, and purulent drainage
    3 Edema, fever, and purulent drainage
    4 Pain, erythema, and edema

11. The IV infusion of a hyperosmolar medication has the potential to cause what type of phlebitis?
    1 Physical
    2 Bacterial
    3 Chemical
    4 Mechanical

12. A patient's IV site is assessed, and a red streak is noted over the catheter track. This sign indicates what type of phlebitis?
    1 Mechanical
    2 Physical
    3 Bacterial
    4 Chemical

13. It is important to stabilize a catheter; thus movement of the catheter at the insertion site is minimal. The rationale for this precaution is that excess catheter movement causes trauma that increases fluid production around the catheter, thereby increasing the patient's risk for:
    1 Phlebitis
    2 Electrolyte imbalances
    3 Infection
    4 Infiltration

14. Thrombophlebitis is the combination of:
    1 Inflammation of a vein and oozing of pus
    2 Inflammation of a vein and a blood clot
    3 Blood clot and hypertension
    4 Hypertension and fever

15. Which of the following symptoms would indicate an IV site infection?
    1 Painful, bruised, and swollen
    2 Red, indurated, and drainage
    3 Swollen, hard vein, and vein streaking
    4 Cold, swollen, and painful

CHAPTER 4: Principles of Central Venous Therapy

1. What is the name of the central vein that leads to the heart and into which most central venous catheters are threaded?
   1 Basilic vein
   2 Superior vena cava
   3 Internal jugular
   4 Axillary vein

2. Which of the following veins is a recommended and common insertion site for a PICC?
   1 Right innominate
   2 Basilic vein
   3 Iliac vein
   4 Subclavian vein

3. Which of the following catheters requires only saline as a flush and not heparin?
   1 Single lumen
   2 Triple lumen
   3 Valved
   4 Open tip

4. Which of the following is a type of long-term catheter?
   1 Implanted port
   2 18-gauge peripheral IV for KVO infusions
   3 Butterfly IV
   4 21-gauge angiocath

5. Which of the following is a disadvantage of a tunneled catheter?
   1 Easy to repair
   2 Able to draw blood samples
   3 Multiple lumens
   4 Altered body image

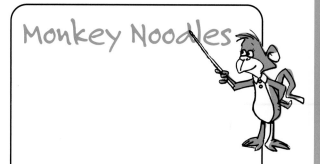

Monkey Noodles

6. Once a Huber needle has been inserted into the port septum, the wings should not point in which direction?
   1 Toward the patient's armpit
   2 Toward the patient's shoulder
   3 Inward toward the patient's sternum
   4 Down toward the patient's chest

7. Mr. Wong is a 26-year-old Asian man who has had an implanted port inserted into his upper-right chest 30 minutes earlier. The physician prescribes chemotherapy to begin as soon as possible. Before beginning chemotherapy, what must **first** be done?
   1 Change the dressing.
   2 Obtain an extension set.
   3 Clean the skin with alcohol.
   4 Obtain a positive blood return from the port to confirm port function.

8. Which of the following is most appropriate for a PICC placement?
   1 A patient with head and neck cancer
   2 An alcoholic patient with seizures
   3 A combative psychiatric patient
   4 An elderly patient with early dementia and no caregiver

9. Site care for a PICC includes a major nursing intervention to prevent phlebitis. This intervention is the:
   1 Application of cold at the PICC site
   2 Application of heat to the upper arm with the PICC site
   3 Raising of the extremity that has the PICC above the heart for 2 hours per day
   4 Application of a compression stocking on the extremity that has the PICC for 2 hours per day

10. Mrs. Smith has an implanted port in her upper-right chest. Her port should be accessed with a:
    1 3-inch syringe needle
    2 Half-inch butterfly needle
    3 Huber needle
    4 16-gauge angiocath

11. The use of a transparent dressing over a CVC insertion site has the following advantage:
    1 Poor visibility of site
    2 Barrier to moisture
    3 Uncomfortable
    4 Increases IV flow rates

12. When preparing a CVC site for Huber needle insertion, a 4-inch diameter area should be swabbed using what type of motion?
    1 Horizontal
    2 Vertical
    3 Circular from outside to inside
    4 Circular from inside to outside

13. Which one of the following factors influences the pounds per square inch (psi) generated by a syringe?
    1 Weight of the patient
    2 Height of the patient
    3 Size of the syringe
    4 Large-bore patent catheter

14. Hemolysis of blood can occur during blood draws from a CVC because of which of the following:
    1 Using a needle that is too big
    2 Gently rocking the filled tube
    3 Drawing blood too rapidly
    4 Using a syringe

15. Anxiety can cause a systemic vasomotor effect that makes removal of a venous access device difficult because anxiety can cause:
    1 Venous spasm
    2 Arterial constriction
    3 Hypotension
    4 Alopecia

CHAPTER 5: Central Venous Catheter Complications

1. Types of common central line complications include all of the following **except:**
   1 Occlusion
   2 Infiltration
   3 Venous thrombosis
   4 Infection

2. Signs and symptoms of impending catheter occlusion are:
   1 Pain
   2 Redness at the insertion site
   3 Inability to aspirate blood
   4 Properly infusing solution

3. Failure to release a clamp is a type of:
   1 Symbolic obstruction
   2 Mechanical obstruction
   3 Singular obstruction
   4 Obstructive atresia

4. Mr. Smith presses his call button complaining of shortness of breath. The nurse hurries into his room and notices that his IV is disconnected. The next action will be to:
   1 Think for a few minutes.
   2 Clamp the catheter.
   3 Turn the patient onto his left side.
   4 Immediately clamp the IV device while rolling the patient onto his left side.

5. Signs and symptoms of CVC local infection include:
   1 Fever, chills, drainage, and malaise
   2 Fever, chills, and anxiety
   3 Redness at the insertion site with drainage
   4 Purple discoloration of the skin 10 cm around the site

6. The most effective way to prevent an air embolus when changing tubing or opening the system is to have the patient perform:
   1 The Allen test
   2 The Swift maneuver
   3 A makeover test
   4 The Valsalva maneuver

7. A malpositioned catheter is
   1 When the insertion site is red and swollen
   2 When the terminal tip of the catheter stays the same
   3 When the terminal tip of the catheter moves out of optimal position
   4 When the catheter will not thread

8. The triad of Virchow applies to what complication?
   1 Venous thrombosis
   2 Cancer
   3 Infection
   4 Air emboli

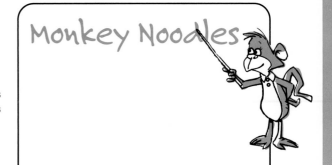

Monkey Noodles

9. Air emboli in conjunction with CVCs can be prevented by all the following **except:**
    1 Teaching the patient about management of the CVC
    2 Using clamps when changing tubing or injection caps
    3 Allowing the patient to take deep breaths when changing tubing
    4 Instructing patient in the Valsalva maneuver (if medically appropriate) when discontinuing a CVC

10. Flushing with a 1-cc syringe against minor resistance can result in _____ _____.

11. Types of solutions used to clear drug buildup or precipitates include:
    1 Blood or iodine
    2 ETOH or hydrochloric acid
    3 Rubbing alcohol or hydrogen peroxide
    4 Sodium phosphate or potassium phosphate

12. Flushing methods to prevent occlusion are:
    1 Power flushing
    2 Brush technique
    3 Turbulent push-pause flushing
    4 Persistent pressure training

13. Types of CVC occlusion are:
    1 Topical (internal and central)
    2 Mechanical (auditory and sensory)
    3 Mechanical (drug and blood)
    4 Mechanical (drug and central)

14. Vancomycin reconstituted has pH denoting:
    1 Acid
    2 Base
    3 Incompatible
    4 Blood cell

15. Infusing a drug with a high pH immediately after infusing a low-pH solution causes:
    1 Drug precipitate
    2 Catheter collapse
    3 Thrombosis
    4 Chemical phlebitis

CHAPTER 6: Pediatric Patient

1. Which of the following statements is **true** regarding the parents' role in the venipuncture procedure?
    1 The parents should perform the venipuncture.
    2 The parents should assist with wiping the site with alcohol.
    3 The parents should be there for support if they choose.
    4 The parents should attach the IV tubing to the IV hub to show enthusiasm.

2. Select the child who should not have his or her telephone conversations interrupted to place an IV.
    1 Toddler
    2 Preschooler
    3 School-age child
    4 Adolescent

3. Keeping the "bits and pieces" away from which group of children is an important safety consideration?
    1 Infants
    2 Preschoolers
    3 School-age children
    4 Adolescents

4. Cold stress is a hazard for small babies, which complicates IV placement because:
    1 Babies experience vasoconstriction.
    2 Babies begin to burn blue carbohydrate stores.
    3 As a result of fat metabolism, the child becomes alkalotic.
    4 Babies experience vasodilation.

5. Grandma Kelly is staying with baby Bryan in the hospital while her daughter works. Her daughter must work because she has the insurance coverage for herself and her children. The older children are in school, and grandma and mom trade places after work, with grandma going home to care for the older children and mom staying with baby Bryan at night. This situation has been particularly stressful for the family. Baby Bryan now needs an IV after a day of fitful crying and outbursts. Grandma insists on accompanying baby Bryan to the treatment room for his IV placement. What is the best way to handle this situation?
    1 Invite grandma to take a break and have a cup of coffee.
    2 Insist that grandma wait in the playroom.

3 Tell grandma if she would like to take a break, she may do so.
4 Tell grandma that the IV can be restarted later, and allow her to spend some unencumbered moments with baby Bryan, holding and rocking him in the rocking chair.

6. What type of approach makes venipuncture easier in young children who usually get very animated after the stylet pierces the skin?
1 Indirect
2 Bevel down
3 Direct
4 Slow

7. A reasonable pattern for assessing pediatric IVs should be:
1 Every 1 to 2 hours
2 Every 8 hours
3 In accordance with parenteral wishes
4 At the patient's discretion

8. The general standard for catheter selection for a child is to use:
1 The largest catheter possible
2 The smallest catheter possible
3 Always a 20-gauge catheter
4 A PICC line for all infants

9. How many attempts should a nurse make to start or restart an IV in a pediatric patient?
1 One
2 Two
3 Four
4 Five

10. IV fluids should be infused using an electronic pump or controller in pediatric patients to prevent:
1 Fluid overload or speed shock
2 Hypertension and dehydration
3 Hyperglycemia and sepsis
4 Paralytic ileus and pancreatitis

CHAPTER 7: Older Adult Patient

1. IV therapy delivered to the older adult requires special attention because of which of the following?
1 Altered immune function
2 Altered gonadal function
3 Altered pituitary function
4 Altered hair growth

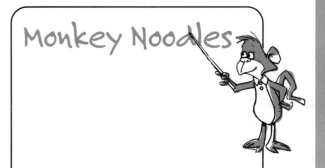
Monkey Noodles

2. The elderly population is projected to:
   1 Remain consistent for the next 20 years
   2 Decrease significantly over the next 20 years
   3 Increase significantly over the next 20 years
   4 Be inconclusive

3. A major physiologic change that occurs during the aging process is:
   1 Loss of epidermis and dermis cells
   2 Increase in subcutaneous tissue
   3 Increase in skin elasticity
   4 Increase in the number of cerebellar brain cells

4. The dosages of medications delivered by IV to an older adult are affected by the normal changes that occur in:
   1 The kidneys and gastrointestinal tract
   2 The liver and gastrointestinal tract
   3 The kidneys and liver
   4 The gastrointestinal tract and circulation

5. The best angle for penetration when inserting an IV catheter into the skin of an older person is:
   1 45 degrees
   2 20 degrees
   3 15 degrees
   4 5 to 10 degrees

6. Vein walls:
   1 Have less collagen in old-old patients, making them susceptible to tearing
   2 Have less smooth muscle, allowing them to easily dilate
   3 Have more smooth muscle, making them less elastic
   4 Are about the same as any adult

7. A central line insertion site on an older patient is assessed, and the patient is found to be lethargic and slightly disoriented. On the food tray on the over-the-bed table, only a small amount of food has been eaten. What happens next?
   1 The patient is awakened, and attempts are made to feed him or her some of the food from the tray.
   2 These symptoms are identified as early signs of infection.
   3 The central line dressing is determined to be dry and intact, and the nurse leaves the room.
   4 The nurse leaves the room without performing the site inspection because he or she does not want to disturb the patient.

8. When inserting an IV catheter in the older patient:
   1 Apply more force to enter the skin of the underarm to make sure to get into the vein.
   2 If the vein is missed, move the catheter around under the skin until the vein is entered.
   3 Avoid excess manipulation of the catheter or "digging" for the vein.
   4 Apply the tourniquet tightly to improve vein visibility.

9. When protecting peripheral IV sites with the elderly patient, the recommended approach is to:
   1 Apply flexible elastic mesh dressing.
   2 Obtain a soft gauze roll and wrap the arm.
   3 Apply wrist restraints to prevent the patient from pulling out the IV.
   4 Verbally remind the patient every 2 hours to protect the IV site.

10. To avoid the occurrence of circulatory overload, the rates of rehydration or IV fluid administration (to a person over the age of 65) would be ideally no more than:
    1 30 cc/hr
    2 50 cc/hr
    3 80 to 100 cc/hr
    4 125 to 150 cc/hr

CHAPTER **8:** Community-Based Infusion Therapy

1. A telephone is most important for home infusion patients for which of the following reasons?
   1 To establish communication with the service provider
   2 To have access to 911 emergency service
   3 To schedule appointments with the home health care nurse
   4 To arrange for delivery of necessary medical supplies

2. _____ is necessary to provide a safe environment to perform procedures.

3. To teach caregivers about home infusion, the first basic principle that needs to be explained and demonstrated is:
   1 To observe a return demonstration
   2 The difference among different types of infusions
   3 How the ingredients in the infusion are to be given
   4 The difference between "sterile" and "clean"

4. When puncturing any item with a needle, the caregiver must first:
   1 Wash the item with antibacterial soap and rinse with sterile water.
   2 Wipe the item with alcohol.
   3 Prepare a cap that will cover the puncture site.
   4 Decide if the item is clean or sterile.

5. The caregiver demonstrates understanding to the nurse by doing what?
   1 Verbalizing the procedure steps, and performing a full return demonstration
   2 Actively listening while the provider gives thorough explanations
   3 Writing a list of questions for the provider
   4 Taking notes provided via the telephone from the provider

6. Instructions for the caregiver should include a _____ _____ of items necessary for the care to be provided, as well as step-by-step instructions.

7. The caregiver should notify the provider of the following signs and symptoms **except:**
   1 Pain or swelling at the infusion site
   2 Chills and fever
   3 Infusion complete
   4 Nausea and vomiting

8. The provider's _____ _____ must always be prominently displayed.

9. The two most important components necessary to identify whether a patient is a candidate for home care are _____ and _____.

10. The home care nurse has more additional activities than an acute care setting nurse. They include all of the following **except:**
    1 Calling and making an appointment with the patient
    2 Coordinate the delivery of all supplies to the patient's home
    3 Secure adequate lighting
    4 Secure all pets so that the work area cannot be contaminated

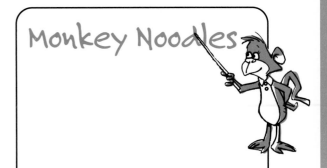
Monkey Noodles

NCLEX CHAPTER *1* ANSWERS

1.3   An advantage of glass is that it is inert. Medications cannot degrade glass; however, some medications can degrade plastic. Disadvantages of glass containers include their heavy weight and bulk, as well as the fact that they are easily breakable. Plastic is light, easy to store, and not easily broken.

2.2   Insulin is best administered using a glass container. Insulin sticks to the walls of a plastic container. D_5W is an IV solution that can be supplied in either glass or plastic containers. Cimetidine and gentamycin do not interact with plastic containers.

3.1   Plastic does not need to be vented because atmospheric pressure on the outside of the bag forces the fluid to flow. Semirigid containers require a vented set to empty completely. Glass containers require a vented set to achieve fluid flow. IV containers are not made of stainless steel.

4.3   Pooling of fluid indicates damage to the bag. It should not be hung. Altering the infusion rate or infusate volume does not affect contamination.

5.3   Placement of the bag 36 inches above the patient's heart is optimal for gravitational systems. Hanging the solution even with the heart would not exert sufficient psi to promote flow. Placing the bag only 12 or 24 inches above the heart would not exert sufficient psi to maintain the prescribed flow rate.

6.4   The components of an administration set are the spike, drop orifice, drip chamber, tubing, and clamp. An end syringe is not part of an administration set. Membrane filters and stopcocks are add-ons.

7.2   The drop orifice determines the size and shape of the drops. The drops are counted to determine the flow rate. The spike punctures the bag. A secondary set is the type of administration set that is used with piggybacks. A clamp is open or closed to regulate flow.

8.2 $(10 \times 120) \div 60 = 20$ drops per minute

9.4   A Leur lock connector screws onto the IV catheter. It does not require force. A slip connector does not screw onto the catheter; it pushes into the catheter. It requires force. A clamp is used to regulate flow. A back-check valve is located on the tubing and prevents fluid from the secondary set from flowing into the primary solution.

10.4   A stopcock is an add-on that is used to determine the direction of flow. A membrane filter is a common end filter. A screen filter is commonly used with blood products. A depth filter absorbs particles in several layers of randomly packed layers.

11.3   Some types of connectors permit the infusion of two or three infusions. Extension sets add length, clamping ability, or both. A depth filter is used to remove particles of a specific size from an infusate. Membrane filters block the flow of specific size particles.

12.3   Gravity systems rely on the height of the solution in relation to the patient's heart (the smaller the distance between them, the slower the rate) to produce enough pressure to achieve the prescribed flow rate. Mechanical systems rely on physical principles such as atmospheric pressure to deliver a prescribed flow rate. Electronic systems rely on electricity, battery packs, or both to deliver a prescribed flow rate. The elastometric pump system is a type of mechanical system and relies on atmospheric pressure to deliver a prescribed flow rate.

13.2   Electronic systems do have free-flow mechanisms. Mechanical, elastometric, and gravity systems do not have free-flow mechanisms.

14.4   The patient's bent wrist is causing an occlusion. The preset psi limit has been surpassed. A low battery signal tells the nurse to plug the pump into an electrical outlet. An air-in-line signal indicates that air is in the line. The door ajar signal indicates that the door of the pump is not properly closed.

15.2   First move and readjust the roller clamp. The tubing under a roller clamp compresses and decreases flow if its position is not changed several times over an 8-hour period. Restarting an IV should only be done after identifying possible problems through a thorough assessment of the IV system. Adding additional resistors or lowering the height of the IV bag will further slow the flow rate.

NCLEX CHAPTER 2 ANSWERS

1.3 A chest x-ray is not needed before peripheral veni-puncture. The patient's mental status can affect site selection, vein stabilization, venous spasm potential, and dressing management. Patient diagnosis can alter venous access. The type of therapy influences vein selection.

2.3 Long-term therapy is longer than 4 weeks. Short-term therapy is shorter than 2 weeks. Intermediate therapy is shorter than 4 weeks. Futuristic is not an IV term.

3.1 Plasma proteins cause vasoconstriction. Plasma pro-teins do not cause vasodilation, heart failure, or chemical phlebitis.

4.3 Patients allergic to latex often have food allergies and should avoid bananas, avocados, tropical fruit, kiwi, or chestnuts. Beef jerky, lettuce, and ice cream do not need to be avoided by patients who are aller-gic to latex.

5.3 C & S needs to be assessed before beginning anti-biotic therapy to ensure that the correct antibiotics are being given to kill the type of bacteria with which the patient is infected. Serum calcium, serum potassium, and prothrombin time will not be altered by administrating antibiotic medications.

6.4 Acetylsalicylic acid (aspirin) increases bleeding time. Its administration places the patient at an increased risk for hematoma formation after venipuncture. Tylenol, garamycin, and digoxin do not alter bleed-ing time.

7.3 A latex-free tourniquet must be used when drawing blood from a patient who is highly allergic to latex. The tourniquet will come in contact with the patient's skin. The disposable syringe and blood tube will not come into contact with the patient. Gauze is latex free.

8.2 Dehydration is directly related to venous distention. The patient's inability to speak will not affect venous distention. Gender and altitude do not affect venous distention.

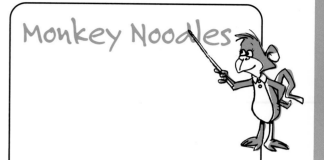

Monkey Noodles

9.1 Use the arm on the opposite side of the mastectomy (left arm) for the peripheral IV. Arms on the side of a mastectomy should be avoided for venipuncture. Feet should also be avoided for venipuncture except in special circumstances.

10.2 The right arm is the functional arm to start an IV. Arms with loss of sensation should not be used for venipuncture. This patient has left-sided paralysis; consequently, the left arm should not be used. The patient requires immediate IV administration. Arterial lines are not used for IV administration.

NCLEX CHAPTER *3* ANSWERS

1.1 It is important to assess the entire IV set-up, insertion site, and dressing regularly, as well as the patient's response, to ensure early detection of peripheral complications. The flow rate is only one part of the IV set-up. Overlooking dressing assessment for integrity may cause complications to be missed. A chest x-ray does not affect peripheral IVs. The IV tubing is only one component of the IV set-up. An assessment of the dressing and the patient's response is crucial. It is important to ask the patient how the IV feels.

2.4 The first response to an occlusion alarm is to assess the entire system for possible constrictions that may be causing increased resistance. Pump malfunction is rare. Restarting the IV should only be performed if it has been determined that the IV catheter is the problem. Heparin infusions require the accuracy and free-flow prevention of an electronic pump.

3.3 Something with the IV catheter must be causing the increased resistance. If the fluid flows freely, then the solution container must be spiked properly, all clamps are open, and no kinks have occurred in the tubing. The diastolic blood pressure does not affect fluid flow. The D_5W solution is free flowing.

4.3 Poor catheter-to-vein ratio can cause infiltration. Good dressing care, good vein elasticity, and low-angle IV insertion technique help prevent infiltration.

5.4 If possible, restart the IV in the opposite extremity, the right ventral upper forearm. If the opposite extremity is not available, then restart the IV at least 3 inches above the infiltration site and on the opposite side of the extremity. An IV should not be restarted below an infiltration.

6.4 Electronic pumps do not sound an alarm for infiltrations. Electronic pumps sound an alarm when the infusion is complete, when an occlusion is detected, or when air in the line has been detected.

7.4 Research has shown that applying compresses does not affect the fluid reabsorption time. Applying dry or moist heat to an infiltration does not affect reabsorption. Cold may decrease pain, but it does not affect reabsorption.

8.2 Amphotericin B is a known vesicant. Dilantin, furosemide (Lasix), and multivitamin solutions are not vesicants.

9.3 Concentrations of 10%, 20%, and 50% dextrose are considered vesicants. D_5W and $D_5^1/2NS$ are not vesicants. Potassium chloride is only a vesicant with high concentrations.

10.4 Pain, erythema, and edema are all symptoms of phlebitis. Cool skin, pain, and swelling might indicate infiltration. Ecchymosis and edema indicate hematoma, and purulent drainage indicates infection. Edema, fever, and purulent drainage may indicate sepsis.

11.3 Chemical phlebitis is caused by solutions that vary significantly from normal blood pH and osmolarity. Physical is not a type of phlebitis. Bacterial phlebitis is caused by bacteria. Mechanical phlebitis is caused by the catheter.

12.1 With mechanical phlebitis, the red streak is over the catheter track. Physical is not a type of phlebitis. Bacterial phlebitis is associated with purulent drainage at the insertion site. The red streak with chemical phlebitis is over the vein track, not over the catheter track.

13.3 Increased fluid is a medium for bacterial growth and infection. Increased fluid production around the catheter does not cause phlebitis. Fluid production does not cause electrolyte imbalances. Leaking fluid is a sign of infiltration, but it is caused by leaking IV solution, not by trauma to the insertion site.

14.2 Inflammation of a vein and a blood clot are both required for thrombophlebitis to occur. Inflammation of a vein and oozing of pus are signs of possible infection. A blood clot is present in thrombophlebitis, but hypertension is not related. Fever is a possible symptom of infection.

15.2 A red, indurated, and draining IV site indicates infection. A painful, bruised, and swollen IV site indicates a hematoma. Swelling, vein streaking, and a hard vein are symptoms of phlebitis. A cold, swollen, and painful IV site indicates infiltration.

NCLEX CHAPTER 4 ANSWERS

1.2 The superior vena cava is the central vein that leads to the heart. The basilic and axillary veins are peripheral veins. The internal jugular connects to the superior vena cava.

2.2 The basilic vein is the recommended and common insertion site for PICCs. The right innominate vein and the subclavian vein are central veins. The iliac vein is not a recommended insertion site for a PICC.

3.3 Valved catheters are designed to require only saline flushes. The determining factor in deciding to flush with saline or heparin is not the number of lumens that a catheter has. Open-tip catheters are not designed to minimize blood reflux.

4.1 An implanted port is used for at least 30 days and up to years and is placed in a central vein. An 18-gauge peripheral IV for KVO infusions, a butterfly IV, and an 22-gauge angiocath are short-term peripheral catheters.

5.4 Altered body image can occur as a result of a tunneled catheter because the catheter is visible externally. Tunneled catheter advantages include ease of repair, the ability to draw blood samples, and its multiple lumens.

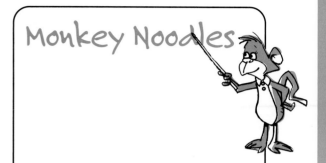
Monkey Noodles

6.1   Rotating the wings toward the patient's armpit promotes needle movement with arm movement and should not be done. Rotating the wings toward the patient's shoulder, inward toward the patient's sternum, or down toward the patient's chest will minimize needle movement.

7.4   A blood return must be obtained to confirm port function before infusing anything. Changing the dressing from surgery, adding an extension first, or cleaning the skin with alcohol is not needed.

8.1   Patients with head and neck cancer are the most appropriate candidates for PICC placement because of surgical and radiation treatment areas. An alcoholic patient or a combative psychiatric patient would most likely not need long-term IV therapy. An older patient without a caregiver would not be able to care for the PICC.

9.2   Heat dilates veins, thereby preventing vein trauma. Cold causes vasoconstriction, which increases potential for vein trauma. Raising the extremity will not enhance venous dilation or venous perfusion. A compression stocking will not enhance venous dilation.

10.3 A Huber needle is a noncoring needle specifically designed for use with a port. Hollow bore needles are not to be used on ports. They core the septum.

11.2 A transparent dressing is a good moisture barrier. Transparent dressings offer excellent site visibility, are comfortable, and help protect the insertion site. Transparent dressings do not affect flow rates.

12.4 Swabbing in a circular motion from inside to outside decreases the potential for contamination of the insertion site. Swabbing horizontal or vertical does not decrease the potential for contamination of the insertion site. Swabbing in a circular motion from outside to inside increases the potential for contamination of the insertion site.

13.3 Syringe size influences psi. Patient weight or height does not affect psi. A large-bore patent catheter has low resistance and therefore will not affect psi.

14.3 A blood draw that is too rapid can cause hemolysis. Using a large needle or syringe and gently rocking the filled tubes decrease the potential for hemolysis.

15.1 Anxiety can cause venous spasm. A PICC is inserted into a vein not an artery. Hypotension is not a symptom of anxiety. Alopecia is the loss of hair.

NCLEX CHAPTER 5 ANSWERS

1.2   Infiltration is a common complication of peripheral catheters, not of central lines. Occlusion, venous thrombosis, and infection are types of central line complications.

2.3   The inability to aspirate blood is an early sign that indicates fibrin build up within a catheter, which may result in a complete occlusion if left untreated. Pain is not associated with impending occlusion. Redness at the insertion may signal site infection. A properly infusing solution is a sign that occlusion is not a problem.

3.2   Mechanical obstructions of IV devices are caused by blockage of the tubing or catheter, which is caused by twisting, clamping, or other physical means. Symbolic obstruction, singular obstruction, and obstructive atresia are all nonsensical terms.

4.4   With air emboli, the first action is to stop the air flow into the catheter by clamping the catheter while positioning the patient on his or her left side. A left-lying position reduces the risk of air blocking the return of blood through the heart, allowing the air to dissipate without fatality. These symptoms signal air embolism. Quick action is required; the nurse does not have a few minutes to stop and think. The longer he or she waits, the more serious the complication will become. Only clamping the catheter will stop the air entry, but clamping does not address the air embolism in the patient's heart. Only turning the patient on his or her left side addresses the air in the patient's heart, but it does not address the continuing inspiration of air with respirations.

5.3   A local site infection is characterized by redness, usually more than 2 cm around the insertion site with drainage. Sometimes, local infections also have tenderness and swelling. Fever, chills, drainage, and malaise are symptoms of sepsis. Fever, chills, and anxiety are not symptoms of infection, but they may indicate symptoms of a more systemic nature. Purple discoloration has no relevance.

6.4 The Valsalva maneuver is the most effective way to prevent air embolus when changing tubing or opening the system. The Valsalva maneuver is a method of holding the breath to prevent pressure changes in the thorax that would encourage air to be sucked into the IV system while open. The Allen's test is for checking arterial blood flow. There is no Swift maneuver. A makeover test is not related to air embolism prevention.

7.3 A change to the terminal tip location of the catheter, out of the SVC or IVC, is considered a malpositioning complication. A red and swollen insertion site indicates local site infection or phlebitis. If the terminal tip location stays the same, no malposition has occurred. In addition, no malposition exists if the catheter cannot be threaded into the body; this instance represents an insertion-related problem.

8.1 The triad of Virchow is a combination of effects that results in coagulation of blood and thrombosis. The triad of Virchow is the combination of injury to the vessel wall and changes in blood flow, which result in stasis and changes in the cell that further causes hypercoagulation. The triad of Virchow does not apply to cancer, infection, or air emboli.

9.3 Allowing a patient to take deep breaths during a tubing change can pull air into the IV system, resulting in an air embolus. It is appropriate to teach the patient about CVC management. Clamps should be used whenever the line is to be open. It is appropriate to instruct the patient to perform the Valsalva maneuver (if medically indicated). This maneuver restricts air passage with changes in intrathoracic pressure during inspiration, reducing the risk of air emboli.

10. Catheter fracture. Pressure applied to a 1-cc syringe will result in high psi, which will fracture a catheter and should not be used for flushing with any CVC.

11.2 ETOH is used to clear lipid build-up within a catheter. Hydrochloric acid is used for low-pH drugs to clear precipitates that have blocked the CVC. Blood is not used for clearing CVCs; it is the cause of obstructions. Rubbing alcohol is not used for clearing CVCs; it is for external use only. Sodium bicarbonate, not sodium phosphate, is used for high-pH drugs to return them to a fluid state with a high pH, thus resolving the precipitate.

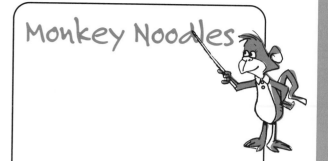
Monkey Noodles

12.3 Turbulent push-pause flushing is a technique used to prevent excess build-up of blood or solutions within a catheter. Power flushing is not used because of the risk of catheter rupture. The brush technique and persistent pressure training have no application for regular CVC maintenance.

13.3 Types of occlusion are mechanical, (drug precipitate and blood). Topical (internal and central) and mechanical (auditory and sensory) are not terms used as types of occlusions. Central is not a type of mechanical occlusion.

14.1 Vancomycin has a pH of 2.4 to 4.5, placing it in the acid range. Incompatible has no application with vancomycin and pH. Acid and base are the only two types of pH.

15.1 Infusing a high-pH solution immediately after a low-pH solution will result in a drug precipitate and potentially catheter occlusion. Collapse of the catheter and thrombosis of the vein will not happen under these circumstances. Chemical phlebitis is a common peripheral complication; it does not occur with central lines.

NCLEX CHAPTER 6 ANSWERS

1.3 Parents should be present only for support and not actually involved in the venipuncture setup or procedure. Parents should never perform or assist with any part of the venipuncture procedure.

2.4 The adolescent is the most in need of privacy, connection to his or her peers, and control of his or her surroundings. The toddler, preschooler, and school-age child generally do not have telephone conversations.

3.1 Infants are very likely to pick up small pieces of supplies and equipment and place them in the mouth, which may provide an aspiration hazard. The sheets and bedding should be double checked to protect these infants from this hazard.

4.1 Brown-fat metabolism produces ketones that lead to acidosis and vasoconstriction. Vasoconstriction complicates IV placement. Brown-fat, not blue carbohydrate stores, is metabolized. The result of the brown-fat metabolism is vasoconstriction, not alkalosis. Infants do not experience vasodilation.

5.4 The IV insertion is not critical. This caregiver has had an exhausting day with this child and has an even more stressful time awaiting her when she returns home to care for the older children. This respite would be good for her and for baby Bryan. Excluding the grandmother from the venipuncture procedure should be a mutual decision between her and the nurse.

6.1 Using an indirect approach makes venipuncture easy in young children who usually get very animated after the stylet pierces the skin. A stylet should always have the bevel up for insertion. When a child is animated, it may be difficult to approach the vein directly on top of it because it might be a moving target. Insertion into the vein should be accomplished as quickly as possible.

7.1 Most facilities require a 1- to 2-hour documented IV check pattern. Less frequent IV site checks can result in late identification of complications. IV checks are mandated by institution policy, not parental or patient wishes.

8.2 The INS recommends using the smallest catheter in the largest vein that will accommodate the prescribed therapy. Using the largest possible catheter will predispose the patient to infiltration or phlebitis. The selection of a peripherally inserted central catheter is dependent on many variables and is not the standard selection.

9.2 After two unsuccessful attempts to restart an IV, the child needs to rest. Because only two attempts are possible at a time, the importance of carefully assessing the veins before insertion is clear. It is important to limit the number of unsuccessful attempts to avoid traumatizing the patient.

10.1 Fluid overload or speed shock are best prevented by using electronic pumps to regulate IV fluids because these pumps have free-flow prevention. Dehydration, sepsis, and pancreatitis do not occur as a result of administering IV fluids.

NCLEX CHAPTER 7 ANSWERS

1.1 Normal physiologic changes occur with aging, which affect the skin, veins, immune system, liver, and kidneys. Gonadal function, pituitary function, and hair growth do not affect IV therapy.

2.3 The geriatric population is increasing and will continue to do so for the next 15 to 20 years.

3.1 A loss of epidermis and dermis cells occurs with aging. A loss of subcutaneous tissue, skin elasticity, and number of cerebellar brain cells occurs, not an increase.

4.3 The reduction in oxidation of enzymes will create a prolonged drug level in the bloodstream. The projected drug half-life will be lengthened. The lack of protein-binding sites in the plasma will create more free drug in the blood. The kidneys and liver are responsible for the majority of drug clearance from the body; their reduced function will slow drug clearance rates. The gastrointestinal tract does not play an important role in affecting drug and blood levels or excretion.

5.4 Lowering the angle on the IV device to approximately 5 to 10 degrees is the best recommendation. This angle accommodates the loss of subcutaneous tissue and lessened resistance of the skin. A 45-, 20-, or 15-degree angle will increase the potential for penetrating the back wall of the vein during venipuncture.

6.1 With advancing age, the connective tissue is reabsorbed and the vein is weakened, making it more easily torn by the introduction of a catheter. The vein wall has less smooth muscle, making the vein less elastic as it ages. The vein wall changes with advancing age.

7.2 The first symptoms of infection are usually lethargy, slight confusion, disorientation, loss of appetite, or any combination of these. Do not attempt to feed the patient. He or she is not asleep, simply lethargic and slightly disoriented. Assessing the central line is appropriate, but identifying the symptoms that are important and require further investigation is necessary.

8.3 Avoiding excess manipulation of the catheter or "digging" for the vein is especially important in the midinner forearm area because of the presence of nerves, tendons, and other structures that can be damaged. Force should never be applied to enter the skin, especially in older patients. Moving around under the skin is painful and can damage nerves, tendons, and other structures; it should not be done. Tourniquets should be applied loosely to prevent overextension of the veins and to protect the skin from tearing and bruising.

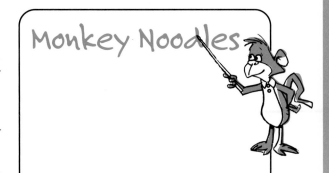
Monkey Noodles

9. 1 Flexible elastic mesh dressing may be easily removed for site inspection; it is not restrictive and will allow for full range of motion of the patient's hand or arm. Wrapping an IV site with a gauze roll of any type is strongly discouraged and is against national standards for IV practice. The insertion site is obscured, preventing site observation and causing injury. Protecting the IV insertion site is more appropriate than taking measures to keep the patient from pulling out an IV. Site protection is a nursing responsibility.

10. 3 Because there is a decrease in the number of nephrons in the kidneys of a healthy older adult, a rate of 80 to 100 cc/hr is sufficient and should not cause fluid overload. A rate of 30 ml/hr or 50 ml/hr are slow KVO rates. A rate of 125 to 150 ml/hr is too fast a rate for the kidneys to accommodate.

NCLEX CHAPTER *8* ANSWERS

1. 2 Access to 911 emergency service is the most important reason for having a telephone. Establishing communication with the service provider, scheduling appointments with the home health nurse, and ordering medical supplies are other advantages of a telephone but are not its most important uses.

2. Electricity is necessary to provide a safe environment to perform procedures. Electricity provides lighting for procedures and refrigeration for the IV solutions.

3. 4 Explaining the difference between "sterile" and "clean" is important to minimize the chance of contamination. Observing a return demonstration of the procedure is part of the fourth basic principle of home infusions. The patient and caregiver do not need to know the differences among different types of infusions. It is only important for the patient or caregiver to understand the solutions that are to be infused. An explanation of how the ingredients in the infusion are to be given is part of the third basic principle of home infusions.

4. 2 The caregiver must first cleanse the item to be punctured with alcohol. Alcohol is the preferred cleansing agent, not antibacterial soap. The area to be punctured must be cleaned before entry, not covered. All injection ports must be cleaned before entry.

5. 1 Although people learn in different ways, a return demonstration is the best way to ensure that a procedure is understood. Information is learned by actively listening to the provider, but it does not demonstrate that learning has taken place. Writing a list of questions for the provider is important and may improve understanding, but it does not demonstrate that learning has taken place. The nurse must see the return demonstration.

6. Instructions for the caregiver should include a written list of items necessary for the care to be provided, as well as step-by-step instructions.

7. 3 Infusion complete is not a sign or symptom; it is not necessary to report infusion complete. Pain or swelling at the infusion site, chills, fever, nausea, and vomiting are symptoms that must be reported to the provider.

8. The provider's telephone number must always be prominently displayed. The patient must have easy access to this number, 24 hours a day.

9. The two most important components necessary to identify whether a patient is a candidate for home care are the home environment and caregiver. Both components are necessary to ensure that therapy can be safely provided.

10. 3 All nurses in all settings must secure adequate lighting before performing IV procedures. This may be a challenge in the home setting. The home care nurse must call and make an appointment and must coordinate the delivery of all supplies. Pets must be secured away from the work area. The acute care setting nurse is not expected to make appointments, coordinate delivery of supplies, or secure pets.

Index

Page references followed by "f" indicate figures and "t" indicate tables.